EXPLAINING MENTAL ILLNESS

Sociological Perspectives

Baptiste Brossard and Amy Chandler

BRISTOL
UNIVERSITY
PRESS

First published in Great Britain in 2022 by

Bristol University Press
University of Bristol
1–9 Old Park Hill
Bristol
BS2 8BB
UK
t: +44 (0)117 374 6645
e: bup-info@bristol.ac.uk

Details of international sales and distribution partners are available at bristoluniversitypress.co.uk

© Bristol University Press 2022

British Library Cataloguing in Publication Data
A catalogue record for this book is available from the British Library

ISBN 978-1-5292-1504-5 hardcover
ISBN 978-1-5292-1505-2 paperback
ISBN 978-1-5292-1506-9 ePub
ISBN 978-1-5292-1507-6 ePdf

The right of Baptiste Brossard and Amy Chandler to be identified as authors of this work has been asserted by them in accordance with the Copyright, Designs and Patents Act 1988.

All rights reserved: no part of this publication may be reproduced, stored in a retrieval system, or transmitted in any form or by any means, electronic, mechanical, photocopying, recording, or otherwise without the prior permission of Bristol University Press.

Every reasonable effort has been made to obtain permission to reproduce copyrighted material. If, however, anyone knows of an oversight, please contact the publisher.

The statements and opinions contained within this publication are solely those of the authors and not of the University of Bristol or Bristol University Press. The University of Bristol and Bristol University Press disclaim responsibility for any injury to persons or property resulting from any material published in this publication.

Bristol University Press works to counter discrimination on grounds of gender, race, disability, age and sexuality.

Cover design: blu inc
Front cover image: Adil Chelebiyev – alamy.com
Bristol University Press use environmentally responsible print partners.
Printed and bound in Great Britain by CMP, Poole

Contents

Acknowledgements		iv
Introduction: Towards a Critical Renewal of the Sociology of Mental Health		1
1	Social Positions 'and' Mental Disorders	9
2	Society as Stressor	34
3	The Weight of Labels	64
4	The Uses of Culture	90
Conclusion: Explaining the 'Mental Health Crisis'		117
Notes		135
References		140
Index		188

Acknowledgements

Of course, the work we present in this book has been nurtured by many, more or less formal, conversations. It contains many insights from many people we cannot cite nor remember. Thus we can only note the most visible interventions. At first, the preliminary reflections underlying this book were outlined in a book chapter co-written by Baptiste Brossard and Florence Weber (2016), '"Folie" et société: ce qu'apporte et ce que manque la question du handicap'. Further ideas were 'collected' and elaborated on the occasion of various gatherings: the mental health section of the 2018 Australian Anthropological Society conference in Canberra, co-organised with Julia Brown; the seminar 'The Social Production of Mental Health' virtually held at the Australian National University in 2020 and 2021, co-convened with Natalie Hendry; and the seminar 'The Social and Cultural Dimensions of Mental Disorders' that also took place virtually in Paris, co-organised with Isabelle Coutant, Frank Enjolras, Ivan Garrec and Javiera Coussieu-Rejes. Let us add to these two joint presentations of our books on self-injury at the Society for the Study of Symbolic Interaction meeting in Lancaster (UK) in 2018, and at the Australian National University School of Sociology, also in 2018 – both were animated by Celia Roberts. May all our collaborators receive our gratitude! In the last stages of writing, we benefited from the feedback and encouragement of Estelle Carde, Bruce Cohen and Florence Weber, while Ian 'Bill' Lucas helped us with our references. At Bristol University Press, Shannon Kneis offered us long-term, benevolent support, which was greatly appreciated.

Introduction: Towards a Critical Renewal of the Sociology of Mental Health

How do social sciences explain the emergence of mental disorders in societies and in individuals?

For instance, can we understand why and how someone becomes 'schizophrenic', 'hyperactive' or 'borderline'? Can we explain the mechanisms through which 'anorexia', 'autism' and 'anxiety' emerge as major mental health issues? Are we able to grasp the causes of what is now called, in many countries, the 'mental health crisis'?

This book aims to map out how sociologists, but also anthropologists and historians, have developed answers to these questions.

Identifying the theoretical and methodological *reasonings* that underlie social explanations for the emergence of 'mental illness/disorder' since the seminal works of Durkheim (1952 [1897]), Faris and Dunham (1939) and others, we provide a critical overview of these approaches with a view to moving this field forward, and reorganizing it, in particular, to help scholars aligned with the sociology of mental health and illness to better realize the promise of this arena of research.

Turning points

There are several reasons why we decided to write this book. Each of us had worked for some time as sociologists researching issues often categorized as relating to 'mental illness'. We both started with studies of self-injury (Chandler, 2016; Brossard, 2018), before moving into broader areas including suicide, dementia and addictions, as well as teaching courses addressing mental health from sociological perspectives. Through these different engagements we became aware of significant challenges in these fields, and of some stagnation. We saw untapped opportunities for sociology and cognate disciplines to contribute more extensively to understandings of and – crucially – *explanations* for 'mental illness'.

Why 'explaining'? This word, in some sociological circles, has a Durkheimian connotation; in others it is associated with the notion of identifying particular 'factors' that can explain mental illness. In our case, we employ it in the broad sense of describing and analysing the processes through which mental disorders come into existence.

This choice reflects a certain intellectual context. Indeed, we stand at the middle of important social, political and epistemological shifts that question what it means to study mental health from a social perspective. These shifts challenge the role that social scientists can uphold in studying mental health. They may constitute opportunities for significant advances to take place, provided, however, that we reflect fundamentally upon our own limitations and potentialities.

First, what is the sociology of mental health concerned with? The multiplication of categories designating mental health issues, the extension of their scope, the management of these issues beyond psychiatry and psychology, as well as what could be called an emotional or psychological turn in our societies, mean that most of us are likely to experience such problems at some point in our lives (Rose, 2018). Mental ill-health is no longer the realm of a minority of marginal individuals, locked in marginal institutions. Mental health conditions enable many people 'in the community' to make sense of and position themselves in their lifeworld. The associated categories seem to resonate with people, 'deep inside', beyond the direct influence of professionals. As a consequence, the sociology of mental health is no longer the sociology of a minority, whose repression tells us something about society and power at large.

Instead, *the sociology of mental health became a sociology of the majority* – the 'general population' epidemiologists talk about – and by extension a *generalized* mode of understanding emotions, norms, behaviours and differences. In this regard, although mental health research has stabilized as a sub-division of health research, the sociology of mental health might be re-considered instead as a fraction of political sociology (in the broadest meaning of the political) or, simply, *sociology*, exploring ways of living together through certain relations of power and emotions.

Second, what is the 'critical' take that sociology can bring to the arena of mental health? Psychiatric power has changed. It is not quite the same authoritarian institution oppressing people by dispossessing them of their fundamental rights anymore, although coercive practices certainly still exist. The deinstitutionalization movement and the 'humanization' of services have changed the game, partly. Today most mental health professionals find themselves in this tension between empowering and controlling patients, what Morrall (2000; and Muir-Cochrane, 2002) call the 'psychiatric paradox'. Those generations of scholars who discovered mental health via Goffman or Foucault, and their dramatic exposures of the domination psychiatry exercised over populations, must adapt to a seemingly benevolent mental health sector from which many users desperately seek help.

Further, psychiatry became the visible tip of the iceberg as professions such as psychologists, social workers, counsellors and therapists of many kinds have taken major stakes in this domain; along with numerous other actors involved in discussing and regulating the mental health of contemporary subjects, from lawyers to teachers. This *mental health apparatus* – the set of institutions, actors, knowledges and discourses that interact to manage certain emotions and behaviours deemed pathological or unhealthy – can certainly still be understood as a political project, deploying norms and forms of control, but perhaps in a less straightforward fashion than when the fundamentals of our disciplines were constructed. This calls, again, for an expansion of the sociology of mental health beyond the wall of hospitals, and even beyond the frame of psy-discourses.

Third, what does 'explaining' mean in this context? We are in a somewhat contradictory situation from an epistemological standpoint. On the one hand, disciplines which traditionally possessed the social legitimacy to address the causality of mental disorders have had to moderate their claims. Research in biomedicine, genetics and neuroscience has still yet to identify clearly cut biomarkers, genes or brain dysfunctions at play in the genesis of mental disorders (Pickersgill, 2011; Rose, 2019; Davies, 2021). In response, the inclusion of 'social factors' are proposed as a minimal way of filling this gap. For instance, 'environmental factors' might 'mediate' the emergence of mental disorder, explaining why neat or causal factors are so difficult to identify (Rapp, 2011). However, as Rose (2018, p 109) asserts about neurosciences – a statement we extend to psychiatry and psychology – it will take more than 'gestural references to the "environment"' to produce actual interdisciplinary perspectives, or a critical complementarity between disciplines that would require manifold cross-disciplinary 'translations' (Brossard and Sallée, 2020).

It is worth noting that a growing minority of professionals substantially consider the social dimensions of mental health: regretting that 'psychiatrists need a social imagination' (Blazer 2005, p 135). Blazer (2005) calls for a 'revival of social psychiatry' (p 183); psychiatrist and anthropologist Enjolras (2016) develops a dual analysis of psychiatric work as both clinical and social, taken as distinct but complementary aspects of care; some psychologists go from placing social factors at the core of their analysis (Cruwys et al, 2014) to proposing psychology be merged into social science (Guerin, 2021).

On the other hand, in the social sciences, we have learned to express caution, if not distrust, regarding causal explanations. Instead, we have at best 'styles of causal thought' (Abend et al, 2013). Decades of constructivism, rightly so, have socialized many of us into thinking that we only explore the surface of disorders, the discourses they trigger, or institutional responses – their social coating, so to speak. But in fact, hundreds of sociological, anthropological and historical works demonstrate the great likeliness that mental disorders have social origins, even when they do not present their argument as a causal one. Further, conceptualizations of 'sociology at the individual level' (Lahire, 2020) facilitate examination of the most intimate realities without necessarily relying on psychological explanations. In fact, most studies of mental health rely on more or less implicit models of why mental illnesses exist, what they are, why they occur in certain contexts. These sometimes 'tacit' aetiologies are at the core of the present book, and articulate several notions of what we mean by focusing on sociological 'explanations' for mental illness.

From this standpoint, epistemological discussions such as that of Hacking (1999) and Rogers and Pilgrim (2014) are helpful. In questioning the traditional opposition between social constructivism, according to which mental disorders do not 'really' exist because they are socially constructed, and realism, according to which mental disorders 'really' exist because they are not entirely a social construction, they enable us to reconsider the status of sociology among other disciplines. This enables us to be *both, and without any contradiction*, critical, for instance contesting the norms conveyed by mental health professionals through their categorizations and work practices, and empathic, acknowledging the real suffering of patients and the relief some might find in receiving professional care. Ultimately, it means that the *social sciences can examine the very production of mental disorders*.

Moreover, not only are we – social scientists – epistemologically *allowed* to attempt to 'explain' mental disorders as much as psychiatrists and psychologists (alongside raising radical doubts regarding the existence and contingency of these disorders), we are also in a situation where our expertise makes particular sense, perhaps more than ever. Thus, the 'mental health crisis' is a textbook example of social fact, offering a compelling and extensive illustration of how societies give human experiences of distress a shape, *and* how they may contribute to the production of this distress in the first place.

Preliminary notes

Before proceeding, we need to clarify some of the vocabulary we will use in this book. Firstly, since we are both sociologists by training, we write more comfortably about 'sociology' as a discipline; however, we will draw on scholarship from anthropologists, historians, geographers, social philosophers and critical psychologists, which we sometimes group under the broad label 'social sciences'. This customary expression does not mean that we endorse a 'scientific' or 'positivist' vision of these disciplines, only that we can identify a common purpose and coherence.

Secondly, we try to regularly specify the countries or cities in which discussed research projects were conducted, noting that, in the literature, research from certain contexts (the US and UK in English-speaking publications, France in French-speaking publications) tends to be presented as naturally generalizable, which can be observed by the absence of mention of the context beyond methodological sections. In contrast, publications originating in studies or from authors in other regions of the world more often present themselves as context-specific, including within their title, and thus implicating context in framing the whole study. Our approach is clear that *all* research is context-specific *while also* bringing a potentiality to be generalized. However, many textbooks talk about 'the sociology of mental health', 'disorders' or 'illness'; while in practice, tending to draw on material relating only or mainly to the US and/or the UK. While we have not entirely shifted away from this tendency, we do try to recognize and problematize this limitation in our own work, as well as in the field of the sociology of mental health.

Third, as in the title of this book, we frame our topic of investigation with the term 'mental illness'. We will also frequently employ others such as 'mental disorder', 'distress', 'troubles', 'issues', or 'disability', both to avoid heavy repetition and to respect how the authors we discuss express themselves. We do want to highlight our reluctance to settle on a particular term or definition. Among the multiple expressions that exist to label this considerable set of emotions and behaviours deemed in some way to be pathological – from schizophrenia to anorexia, to anxiety disorders to autism, and so forth – 'mental illness' seems to be one of the most socially widespread. The term is semantically imperfect (are all of the experiences we discuss necessarily understood as 'illnesses' that are 'mental', all the time? Absolutely not!), and we could spend weeks (and indeed did so while writing this book) disserting about what 'mental', 'illness', 'health' and 'disorder' imply and evoke. We also include work on self-harm and suicide because these are often socially understood as linked to mental health issues (and as noted above, these practices were in some ways our own 'gateways' to the sociology of mental illness). However, we acknowledge the ongoing debates about whether it is appropriate to categorize self-harm or suicide (Marsh, 2010) in terms of mental illness, some of which we have contributed to (Chandler, 2016; Button and Marsh, 2020). Such debates are relevant to a much wider array of 'mental illnesses' and our interest in navigating and interrogating these is what – in part – drives our inquiry.

Minimally, each of these terms loosely relates to some troubles or disruptions attributed to the psychology of people, their mental life or their psyche. *They are only one prism that our societies – following the influence of some groups – use to qualify certain differences among their members.* As these differences become reified through the sustained activities of institutions designed to regulate them (Foucault, 1961), studying 'mental illness' sociologically requires us, *at the same time*, to study the realities these notions point to and to question what they mean. As such, we propose that employing terms such as mental illness and disorder does not negate us retaining a certain distance towards these categories. Importantly, this double movement – studying what labels designate and studying labelling itself – is necessary to a sociology of mental health freed from the opposition between realism and constructivism, one which facilitates our ambitious focus in this book, *explaining mental illness*.

Structure of the book

In writing this book, we chose not to reintroduce the usual theoretical divisions along which many other textbooks are structured, such as those between conflict theories, functionalism and interactionism, or structuralism and post-structuralism. Separating out research into these categories does not capture the wealth of existing academic positions, and tends to lock researchers into a priori theoretical assumptions, rather than spotlighting points of debates and potential improvement. For this reason, we felt the best way to serve the academic community was to focus instead on *reasonings*.

We conducted a broad review of the Anglophone and Francophone academic literature to dissect the methods and rationales at work when social scientists examine the sociogenesis of mental disorders. In these literatures, we distinguished between *reasonings*, whose identification will always be, by definition and to some extent ideal-typical, reductive of the publications which we drew them from. It will always be 'more complicated than that'. Obviously, this is not because we wish to unfairly simplify these works. Rather, we believe that this process, in addition to its pedagogical merits, allows us to gain access to and better discuss the fundamental assumptions on which these works rely, which in turn will foster the generation of critical insights necessary to set out a new agenda for the sociology of mental health and illness.

The four main reasonings we identified are summarized below. Each of these makes up one of the four substantive chapters of this book, while a concluding chapter summarizes our propositions and attempts to apply them to the 'mental health crisis'.

- Mental disorders correspond to forms of *social positioning*, primarily because they are unequally distributed in societies, which suggests that they emerge due to conditions reflecting certain social positions, generally disadvantaged ones. Further, they can be interpreted in light of social stratification (including socioeconomic status but also gender, race, and so forth) in several ways: for example, because they reflect the social divides that structure a given society, and because their very definition often involves targeting and even producing certain populations. In this chapter we argue that the field has stagnated, focusing excessively on correlations rather than explanations. We propose that three alternative approaches – intersectionality, configurational and definitional – can help to reinvigorate sociological work on social positions and mental illness.

- Mental disorders are an outcome of the social production of *'stress'*, because some individuals are exposed to emotional pressure without possessing the resources to deal with these. From this perspective, known as the stress paradigm and quite dominant in US sociology, society generates adversities that generate stress, which might turn into mental disorders. We explore the main working hypotheses of this paradigm before turning to ways that the stress process model might be enhanced, or upended. Firstly, discussing the concept of minority stress, we address how inequalities can be more deeply accounted for in stress studies. Secondly, we propose greater integration between the study of stress and the sociology of emotions; drawing on approaches to anger and paranoia to illustrate this.

- Mental disorders are the by-product of *categorization* processes, because the production of these categories has performative effects, namely, labelling mechanisms partly create the reality that they define. Some classical theories support this argument, especially Scheff's labelling theory but also a significant facet of Foucault's theory of knowledge applied to 'madness'. We review contemporary works on labelling, from medicalization to stigma studies through microsociology, and propose three ways of renewing these perspectives: considering socio-political arrangements at the origin of categories; unpacking performativity in social life; and questioning why diagnoses and labels exist.

- Mental disorders embody reactions to *sociocultural contexts* because their symptoms express – in somewhat distorted fashions – certain features of these contexts. Summarizing some early work that sketched links between culture and mental health, from Mauss to Fanon, we turn to the debates that revolved around the introduction of 'culture-bound syndromes' in the Diagnostic and Statistical Manual of Mental Disorders (DSM)[1] and concerns about the (contested) universality of disorders. This chapter presents several models though which contemporary social sciences attach mental disorders to cultural contexts. Highlighting the necessity of discussing crucial issues, especially the role of colonialism and cultural reductionism, we outline approaches which go further, including rethinking the status of 'madness' in research projects and building integrative models that account for the complexity of 'cultures'.

★★★

To conclude, we hope that this book can be simultaneously read in two ways.

On one hand, it is an *advanced textbook* reviewing the main approaches developed in sociology and neighbouring disciplines to understand the emergence of mental health issues in individuals and societies. Students interested in the sociology of mental health and its contemporary challenges can find an in-depth introduction to this area of reflection.

On the other hand, it is a *critical assessment* of the sociology of mental health, pointing to its limitations and outlining paths to overcome them. Researchers will gain a sense of the most significant debates (according to us) and be presented with a relatively innovative structuration of this field, providing inspiration for further innovation.

If there were one idea to remember from this book, it would be that the current specialization of mental health research within sociology (often as a sub-type of health research) around specific concepts and methods, while allowing for more theoretical accuracy and targeted data collection, runs the risk of losing sight of the *bigger picture*. Mental health is an *embedded* aspect of social relations, organizations, identities and structures. As such, all the chapters of this book conclude with an invitation to consider the sociology of mental health as the sociology of something broader than mental disorders themselves: these disorders are – we argue – not only ways of experiencing the world, marking people who may be treated and labelled by medicine, or a focus of significant and growing research; they can also be seen as providing privileged entry points towards a deeper examination of the social world. Thus, a sociology of mental health need not be sequestered as a sub-section of an existing specialization within sociology: it provides insights relevant for sociology as a whole.

1

Social Positions 'and' Mental Disorders

What is wrong with Madame Bovary? In the novel of the same name, Gustave Flaubert portrays the life of a woman in mid-nineteenth century France. The wife of a rural doctor, Emma Bovary struggles with the limitations of her existence. She invests herself in varied activities, navigating uneven mindsets and emotions, hoping to make sense of mundanity and tackling the boredom of her milieu – the petit bourgeoisie of a small town in Normandy. She tries to be a perfect housewife. She attempts to be a dedicated devotee. She daydreams of affairs. She has affairs. She plays the piano. She supports the professional achievements of her husband. She has problems with her 'nerves'. At least, this is what the men around her imagine. Madame Bovary's changing mood, they assume, is due to her feminine nature. Doctors seek to solve the problem with drugs. Drowning in debts, she kills herself.

This story illustrates a very sociological question. Does the position someone holds in their society influence and/or result from their mental health? In this chapter, we use the term 'social position' as the broadest expression to denote the status and situation individuals hold in their society, including their position in terms of social class but also gender, 'race', geographical residence, age, and so forth. This is a way for us to discuss the field of mental health inequalities taken as a whole, without stumbling upon each conceptual particularity. Manifold studies have demonstrated a 'relationship' between several measures of social position and rates of various mental illnesses: in general, the lower people are in the social hierarchy, the higher their chance of experiencing some mental health-related difficulties. This consistent finding represents a major component in our understanding of the social genesis of mental disorders. It tells us that mental health has *something to do with* social position – but not what.

Indeed, the mechanisms through which such correlation operates remain subject to much debate. Do mental health problems *cause* people to 'drift' to a lower socioeconomic status or do they develop such problems *because of* socioeconomic disadvantages? More fundamentally, why? Let us return to Emma Bovary. Does her situation trigger or result from her 'nerve' issues? Is emotional disturbance a cause, or an outcome? Does she suffer from her status as a woman or as a member of the petit bourgeoisie? Would she experience more weariness if she were a man, from another milieu? Maybe. The point is, posing the problem in such fashion is reductive. Even if we imagine the fictive possibility of a survey that would unveil similarities among all the Emma Bovarys of the world, seeking 'social factors' and 'outcomes' would miss a crucial fact: mental health is lived *through* social positions, and conversely, social positions are lived *through* mental health. These two notions designate realities that overlap and are mutually constructing.

The sociology of mental health, now that it has unveiled significant *correlations*, should focus more on explaining how, and with what effects, such *intertwining* occurs. After critically outlining major findings from the field of mental health inequalities, this chapter charts three broad, emerging perspectives within contemporary research which particularly advance knowledge in this research area. First, *intersectional perspectives* contend that articulating the various features of social position make the study of inequalities and differences more accurate and meaningful, with important implications in relation to oppression, domination and stereotypes. Second, *configurational perspectives* see social position not only as a set of variables interacting with one another but as configurations through which mental health issues are constructed and expressed. Third, *definitional perspectives* suggest that not only are mental health difficulties unequally distributed in societies, but also their very categorization pre-determines the publics to which they shall apply. Ultimately, this chapter revolves around a critique of the 'correlation paradigm' that grounds the majority of works in mental health inequalities and calls for an – already ongoing – renewal of this research question.

Inequalities in mental health: a story of variables?

In mental health research, as in other fields, the study of inequalities has been historically constructed as the research of correlations between, on the one side, elements of social status and, on the other, indicators of mental health. In this section, we review this approach, showing its considerable contributions but also its limitations.

The quest for social determinants

An association between poverty and illness (physical or mental) has been suspected since at least the nineteenth century, with hygienist medicine. However, it is from the 1930s onward, with the first community studies, that this relationship was more seriously established. These early studies found that the highest rates of diagnosed disorders could be observed in the poorest neighbourhoods or among people holding the lowest socioeconomic statuses; and further, that even the types of diagnosed disorders varied with social position.

Faris and Dunham (1939) pioneered an ecological approach to mental disorders in 1930s Chicago, arguing that local social issues – isolation, ethnic conflicts or economic hardship – influenced the mental illnesses people are more likely to suffer from. Two decades later, Hollingshead's team (Hollingshead and Redlich, 1958) defined five classes in a Connecticut town, based on socioeconomic, occupational and geographical criteria, and discovered the same correlations. Upper class patients, although less diagnosed overall, were more likely to be diagnosed with 'neurotic' pathologies (such as depression) while working class patients were more likely to be diagnosed with 'psychotic' pathologies (such as schizophrenia). Studying Manhattan's East Side, Srole and colleagues (1962) included the severity of symptoms in their measurements, and additionally identified differences of mental health depending on forms of social mobility (upward, downward, no mobility). Since the 1960s, thanks to these works often gathering together sociologists and psychiatrists, strong evidence exists that rates and types of mental disorders are unequally distributed in the population. A multitude of studies have built on these preliminary observations.

Since the 1980s, community studies progressively gave way to population studies. Aiming to reach greater statistical authority, the latter favoured representative national samples over pre-existing local communities. In parallel, we can observe a widening of the research objects, moving away from a narrow focus on psychiatric diagnoses, towards increasingly sophisticated attempts to measure degrees of wellbeing or psychological distress. The Epidemiologic Catchment Area Study is an early example of a population study, conducted across a large sample of the US population (in five targeted areas); it covered 20,000 people between 1980 and 1983. Using a composite measure of socioeconomic status combining education, occupation and household income, the survey showed that the rates of most disorders varied depending on socioeconomic status, the poorest people being disadvantaged in all regards. But this disadvantage was not constant. The lower quartile was almost eight times more likely to suffer from schizophrenia than people in the highest quartile. This proportion was 'only' two times for major depression.[1] The US National Comorbidity Study, performed between 1990 and 1992, was the first to use a research diagnostic interview aligned with DSM-III-R (Diagnostic and Statistical Manual of Mental Disorders)[2] categories. This survey found the same correlation between mental disorders and lower socioeconomic statuses, mostly measured with years of education. In the UK, numerous studies have identified similar correlations between (mental) health and socioeconomic status. The Black Report (Townsend et al. 1988) notoriously underlined these inequalities, and subsequent studies, including the Psychiatric Morbidity Surveys, repeat these findings.

In seven words: the poorer the sicker, and vice versa.[3] The steady finding of a negative health gradient in multiple contexts and with multiple methodologies led to the idea that socioeconomic status is a *fundamental cause* of health and mental health (Link and Phelan, 1995; Reiss, 2013).

This idea also set the scene for further research on mental health in several countries, reflecting on macroeconomic processes such as recessions, austerity policies (Antonakakis and Collins, 2014) and welfare regimes (De Moortel et al, 2015), as they shape the structure of opportunities (Coope et al, 2014; Barr et al, 2015) and inequalities (Kangmennaang and Elliott, 2018) on which population mental health relies.

Today, many studies aim to better articulate the link between socioeconomic status and mental health (Aneshensel, 2009). To do so, they resort to three methodological directions: multiplying indicators of social status; seeking the most relevant measurable aspects of status; and integrating relational and subjective aspects. Note that we discretely slid from 'class' to 'socioeconomic status': this vocabulary shift reflects the progressive abandonment of the Marxist-inspired understanding of class as a collective structure in favour of a social stratification approach, which emphasizes the individual level of analysis (Muntaner et al, 2000).

A key approach has been the *multiplication of indicators of socioeconomic status*, in order to better understand what exactly it might be about inhabiting a particular position or class which contributes to poorer mental health outcomes. Examples of combined indicators to account for socioeconomic status (SES) include educational attainment and area of residence (Kim et al, 2010, in South Korea), educational attainment and household per capita expenditure (Lei et al, 2014, in China), or, for children, parental educational attainment, whether their birth was paid for by Medicare in the case of the US,[4] the district of residence's median property value and education level (King and Bearman, 2011). Other possibilities are Owens' (2020) study of attention deficit hyperactivity disorder (ADHD) diagnoses in the US, which measured socioeconomic status with a standardized scale combining parents' educational attainment, their income and the prestige of their occupation, showing that while high-SES children have access to more resources when they are diagnosed, their later school performance is more affected by the diagnosis than low-SES children. Another is Nishimura's (2011) study of depression in Asia, that demonstrates how such indicators are culturally embedded, for instance, employment contracts appeared to matter more in Japan than Korea, where educational attainment was the most significant variable.

Leading from this, other studies seek to *identify the most relevant measures*; which they attempt by isolating specific aspects of SES in order to improve the accuracy of our understanding of mental health inequalities. Among the most commonly addressed factors in various national contexts are: economic uncertainty (Vandoros et al, 2019), financial strain (Bierman, 2014) which may be accompanied by water and food insecurity (Bergmans and Wegryn-Jones, 2020; Maxfield, 2020), problems accessing housing (Kavanagh et al, 2016), debts (Sun and Houle, 2018; Swanton and Gainsbury, 2020), job precarity (Moscone et al 2016; Burgard and Seelye, 2017), high work load (Kamerade et al 2019; Sato et al 2020) and/or poor working conditions (Marchand et al 2005). Additionally, and increasingly focused upon, the social position held in childhood has long-lasting effects on our mental health, as Pryor et al (2019) showed in Denmark. Note that these studies tend to convert abstract measurements of socioeconomic status into tangible difficulties that people living in poverty can experience.

Finally, other studies focus on *relative status*, or *subjective status*, which relates to the opinion someone has about their position. Overall, subjective feelings of deprivation or inferiority are found to be detrimental to mental health (Mishra and Carleton, 2015; Beshai et al 2017). Sometimes the measured effects of subjective social status even exceed that of objective status, as Sakurai et al (2010) suggest about Japanese women whose subjective status indicators are more significantly correlated to psychological distress than 'objective' status indicators such as household income and education. Lee and Kawachi (2017) found that in Korea, socializing with people from a higher position increases the likelihood of experiencing depressive symptoms.

Relatedly, *status incongruence*, that is, the discrepancy between one's status and other aspects of one's life or environment, can be used to develop this approach. This typically happens when someone holds a job whose required skills do not match their educational level or class background. Without surprise, negative status inconsistency – for instance, when someone is or thinks they are over-qualified for their occupation – generally correlates with poorer mental health (Albor et al, 2014; Milner et al, 2017), potentially through the feelings of shame this situation can arouse (Lundberg et al, 2009).

Another set of studies addressing relative status is found in Neo-Marxist approaches which examine the *types of relation generated by modes of production*. This includes attending to managerial domination and ownership (Muntaner et al, 2013), for instance via the concept of 'contradictory class locations' – which is used by Muntaner and collaborators to explain greater rates of depression and anxiety among middle managers, a finding which otherwise contrasts with the more usual gradient of greater distress being concentrated among more disadvantaged groups. Prins et al (2015) argue that those inhabiting supervisory roles (with more power than workers, but less than higher-level managers or business owners) can be understood as inhabiting a contradictory class position, sitting between workers and capitalists; they propose that the incongruence of this position contributes to greater distress – manifesting in higher rates of mental disorder.

Adding more variables

In the last decades, research has drawn in more and more aspects of social position, demonstrating significant correlations with rates of mental distress: race, gender, age, generation, social mobility, migrations, marital status, sexual orientation, social networks, places of residence, and so forth. In the following paragraphs we sketch out some of the major findings in relation to each of these variables.

Disadvantaged racial groups are more likely to suffer from mental health problems (Takeuchi and Williams, 2003), a finding tied to structural racism (Williams, 2018; Shellae Versey et al, 2019; Nazroo et al, 2020), including in psychiatry (Fernando, 2017), broader discrimination (Baert et al 2016; Brown et al 2018) and unequal access to care (Cook et al, 2013). Multiple elaborations on the links between race, mental health and social class have been articulated since the 1980s (Kessler and Neighbors, 1986). However, especially in the US, it is sometimes reported that black people, despite greater life adversities, have similar mental health outcomes to white people (Barnes and Bates, 2017). This finding has been termed the *race mental health paradox*, and might result from under-reporting of mental health issues among African Americans (Alang, 2016), who – according to some studies – express distress in ways not captured by standardized scales. This hypothesis taps into wider doubts regarding the measurement of mental health issues (Takeuchi and Williams, 2003; Rockett et al, 2006) and racist bias in diagnosis. For instance, one study found that UK and US physicians were more likely to attribute physical (endocrinological specifically) causes to depressive symptoms when their patients are black (Adams et al, 2014).

In recent years, this area of work has further expanded. It is increasingly recognized that much greater diversity of racial or ethnic groupings should be examined – moving substantially beyond the black–white dichotomy (Takeuchi and Williams, 2003; Ajrouch and Antonucci, 2018). Others have proposed measuring skin tone instead of racial identity, and thus addressing 'colourism' more specifically (Louie, 2019). In attempting to explain racial disparities in mental health, studies have considered the socializing implications of race (Erving and Thomas, 2017), such as education and early childhood, which may have lasting effects on mental health experience and expression (Becares et al, 2015; Kysar-Moon, 2019); and refining our understanding of racist discrimination and its impact on the mental health of ethnic minorities (Williams, 2018).

Striking mental health differences are observed *between women and men*. Depression rates are much higher in women (Van de Velde et al, 2010; Platt et al, 2020) and this significantly increases with age (Bracke et al, 2020), while suicide rates are much higher in men (Niehaus, 2012; Nowotny et al, 2015). A common argument – also commonly critiqued (Hill and Needham, 2013) – is that women are more likely to suffer from 'internalizing disorders' such as depression and anxiety, while men would struggle more with 'externalizing disorders' such as substance abuse or antisocial behaviour (Rosenfield, 2012; Rosenfield and Mouzon, 2013). Possible explanations include: the effect of traditional gender socialization, such as the legitimation of violence for men and introversion for women (Busfield, 2014, an argument recently re-branded 'self-salience theory', Gibson, 2014, Rosenfield, 2012); the higher vulnerability of women, who hold more social roles than men while enjoying less recognition and opportunities (the 'sex role theory', Gove and Tudor, 1973); and the gendering of the very definitions of mental disorders – see the 'definitional perspective' below.

Qualitative research compellingly recalls the emotional pervasiveness of traditional gender stereotypes in the expression and symptomatology of mental disorders: tough but isolated men (Ridge et al, 2011; Oliffe et al, 2019; Herron et al, 2020) and women torn by guilt, shame, and lack of self-confidence (del Mar García-Calvente et al, 2012; Frieh, 2020; Denneson et al, 2020). Trans and non-binary people are now increasingly recognized and studied, both for the high levels of distress and suicide reported among them and the buffering effects of membership in LGBT+ communities on mental health (Ruth and Santacruz, 2017; Sherman et al, 2020). It is becoming increasingly untenable for researchers to fail to recognize the diversity of gender identities, and how these may impact (aside from traditional studies of binary gender difference) on mental health experiences and outcomes (Chandler and Simopoulou, 2021; Newman et al, 2021).

Marital status has been a long-lasting source of interest among mental health scholars, with the recurrent finding that being married 'protects', statistically speaking, from mental illness. Since Durkheim, this argument has been repeatedly tested from the case of suicide (Kyung-Sook, et al, 2018) to that of mental illness (Lindström and Rosvall, 2012). Disruptions in family life are correlated with poorer mental health (Lu, 2012); therefore, marital stability improves wellbeing. Men, who were benefiting more than women from their marriage (while more affected by its rupture) seem to have lost this statistical advantage in the late twentieth century (Simon, 2002).

Recent research has emphasized higher rates of mental illness, distress, suicide and self-harm among *LGBT+ people* (McDermott and Roen, 2016), attributed to social integration problems (Hsieh, 2014) and exposure to stressful situations (Frost et al, 2017), especially during identity transitions (Everett, 2015). Challenges within this research area include the incorporation of trans people with LGB people – conflating gender and sexuality. Relatedly, the tendency to 'lump together' an incredibly diverse group of people constructed as an at-risk public (King et al, 2008) raises questions as, for instance, rates of self-harm might differ between lesbian, gay and bisexual people, with bisexual women reporting far higher rates of self-harm, as do 'unsure' individuals (Mann et al, 2020). Finally, the public health approach to LGBT+ people may imply that queerness is the 'cause' of distress, whereas alternative perspectives such as those set out by McDermott and Roen (2016), Cover (2012) or the minority stress framework (see Chapter 2; Meyer, 2003) more convincingly highlight how structural and cultural forces shape stigmatizing meanings and responses to sexual and gender minorities.

That certain mental disorders are more likely to be diagnosed in certain *neighbourhoods* constitutes a ground-breaking contribution of the sociology of mental health. The interpretation of this relationship has long been that the neighbourhoods in which people live reflect their socioeconomic condition. However, place includes two distinct components: the population that inhabits a district, and the features of the district itself; both components interact. In his synthesis of community studies results in the US, Kohn (1973, p 157) noted that the larger the city, the stronger the correlation between rates of schizophrenia and social class (which could explain some otherwise contradictory findings). It is now widely acknowledged that neighbourhood statistically 'moderates', in the statistical sense of the term, the weight of other social and social psychological variables on mental health, such as difficult family circumstances (Lima et al, 2010). Furthermore, indicators such as neighbourhood stability (Ross et al, 2000), perceived social cohesion, support and safety (Scott et al, 2018; Ruiz et al, 2019; Miao et al, 2019), possibilities for daily mobility (Vallee et al, 2011; Lowe and DeVerteuil, 2020), employment rate (Curtis et al, 2019), segregation (Lee, 2009) and appreciation of the built environment (Araya et al, 2006) strongly correlate with mental health outcomes. Suicide research holds a singular place in this literature, since suicide clusters can turn a neighbourhood's social cohesion into dangerous ties (Derek Cheung et al, 2014; Cairns et al, 2017).

Another set of approaches delves into the protective effect of *social networks*, *social capital* or *social support*. As for socioeconomic status, there is a movement towards specialization of the indicators, such as network diversity, trust in neighbours (Bassett and Moore, 2013), experience of 'positive' interactions (Laurence, 2019) or involvements in local organizations (Landstedt et al, 2016). Three general findings can be identified. First, social isolation is associated with most mental health problems to the extent that it is suspected of being a primary cause (Almedom, 2005; Song, 2011; Riumallo-Herl et al, 2014). Second, certain types of social capital can moderate pathogenic correlations, for instance between parental stress and children overeating

(Mandelbaum et al, 2020) or socioeconomic status and mental health inequalities (Nielsen et al, 2015). Third, in some cases, connections can also facilitate the 'diffusion' of mental health problems (Guan and Kamo, 2016). Referring to suicide, Baller and Richardson (2009, p 261) called this effect the 'dark side of the strength of weak ties', an issue taken up by Mueller and Abrutyn's (2016) study of suicide suggestion in a cohesive community in the US and by Liu et al (2010) with autism rates in California. These three findings converge in recent quantitative and qualitative research exploring the ambivalent meaning of social ties, providing both happiness and stress, support and judgements (Rice et al, 2011; Huang et al, 2018).

Migration is often associated with mental health issues due to the poor material conditions, stigmatization and trauma that migrants, and especially refugees, go through (O'Donnell et al, 2020). But migration is also known for its *epidemiological paradox*, also called the *immigrant health paradox*. Despite adversity, migrants from non-Western to Western countries report relatively good physical and mental health (John et al, 2012; Montazer and Wheaton, 2017; Gutierrez-Vazquez et al, 2018). As with the 'race mental health paradox', this observation may well be explained by lower declarations among migrants, partly because they would not conceptualize their potential distress in medical terms (Turcios, 2017). Alternative explanations for this paradox suggest migrants may experience relatively better material conditions of life after migration (Barnes et al, 2020), or that the finding is a result of the numerous formal and informal selection processes underlying migration. Importantly, in some national contexts, legitimate fear of apprehension or detainment by authorities may be a significant deterrent to help-seeking and participation in surveys (Duncan, 2015; Fekete, 2020; Mills and Klein, 2021).

Many studies have sought to evaluate how *inter- and intra-generational social mobility* impacts mental health. They have not been conclusive (Fox, 1990; Tiffin et al, 2005). However, the entanglement between mental health and educational attainment – in both ways – now has strong evidence (McLeod et al, 2012; Bracke et al, 2013; Bauldry, 2015). Two opposite hypotheses are considered. First, the theme of pathogenic social mobility, which had its heyday in the 1950s and 1960s, highlights the social and psychological 'costs' incurred by the transgression of class boundaries (Lipset and Bendix, 1959), what is sometimes referred to as 'Sorokin's dissociative thesis'. Second, most contemporary studies prefer the thesis that upward mobility, because it comes with increased economic comfort and social prestige, improves mental health (Chan, 2018; Bridger and Daly, 2020). But research on mobility has gradually shrunk, faced with a lack of clear findings and, perhaps, due to its troubling contrast with the cultural valuation of success and material wealth.

In terms of *age*, prevalence of mental disorders generally follows a U-shape: very prevalent in adolescence and youth, then decreasing over adult life to come back again with old age. But some studies presented data that diverge from the classical U, which questions the usual assumption that adolescence and old age would carry some obvious vulnerability (Butterworth et al, 2006; Bell, 2014). Additionally, age as a stand-alone variable tends to be replaced with the more productive approaches of life course (Schoon and Bynner, 2003; Darin-Mattsson et al, 2018) or of cohorts, that is, historically situated age groups. Cohorts have strong statistical significance in suicide rates (Phillips, 2014), and the effects of economic recessions on mental health can be measured on successive generations (Curtis and Curtis, 2011). Explorations of the generational meaning of mental health and social ties give interesting results. Regarding bipolar disorder in China, Ng (2009) argues that whereas people who grew up during the Mao era are inclined to explain their illness with external circumstances, younger patients emphasize individual responsibility. Investigating two disadvantaged neighbourhoods in Malta, Satariano (2019) shows that the meanings attributed to social capital by different generations differ: adults welcome local connections as forms of social support while teenagers consider them a detrimental influence. As we will see, studies of generations have the potential to empirically tie individuals' mental health to the course of history.

Explanatory models

How do we make sense of all these correlations? Two main explanatory models have long structured the field of possible answers to this question;[5] they also apply to physical health. On the one hand, the *selection hypothesis*, or *social drift hypothesis*, contends that social positions partly result from mental health issues. For instance, if there are higher rates of schizophrenia among poorer people, it is because symptoms of schizophrenia prevent people from accessing work or high paid/status jobs. In this model, income or financial resources are tied to marital status and geographical location: mental disorders make it difficult to get married or get housing in better resourced neighbourhoods. Note that this hypothesis can only apply to variables on which individuals have – in theory – some control: this excludes race. On the other hand, the *causality hypothesis* advances that mental disorders are the result of issues associated with social positions. If we find more schizophrenia diagnosed among the working class, it is because the adversity of existence, material conditions of life and emotional socialization in this class lead more of its members to such a diagnosis. The same can be said of all the above-mentioned variables, whose implications on people's trajectory in life might be understood to *cause* mental disorders.

Today, most researchers agree that both processes overlap (Mulatu and Schooler, 2002; Mossakowski, 2014). The question became how to conceptualize the complex mechanisms through which the mutual influence between mental health and social position operates, which relates to how the latter is *embodied*. We identified five ideal-typical lines of reasoning:[6]

- *Cultural/behavioural explanations:* depending on their social position, people are socialized differently and adopt different lifestyles, which shapes their mental health experiences, and ultimately their lifestyle.
- *Materialist explanations:* depending on their social position, people live in unequal material conditions, and poor conditions of life are detrimental to mental health, which in turn worsens their material situation.
- *Social role/support explanations:* depending on their social position, people hold unequal quantities and qualities of social roles and ties, which conditions their mental health and potential social support, which in turn affects their social integration.
- *Stress explanations*: depending on their social position, people are unequally exposed to stressors conductive to mental disorders and have unequal resources to deal with these (see Chapter 2).
- *Artefact explanations:* depending on their social position, people experience and express their emotions in different manners, which impacts the diagnoses they receive; similarly, professionals have various personal and social 'biases', which impacts the diagnoses they give.

These explanatory models often remain more working hypothesis or theoretical premises than empirically elaborated analyses. Hence in many publications, the methodological tools used to explore the relationships between different variables discretely become ontological assertions: researchers demonstrate a correlation between, say, rates of diagnosed schizophrenia and poverty in a given neighbourhood and *then* look into the reasons of this correlation – maybe it is stress, socialization, material deprivation, and so forth. As a result, underlying a significant body of work in the sociology of mental health lies an overall confusion between correlation and causality. This is the *paradigm of correlation*.

In this paradigm, many projects work with notions such as socioeconomic status, race or gender without paying sufficient attention to the context-dependent nature of these concepts-made-variables. For instance, numerous studies from the US assert that the lower people are in the social hierarchy, the more likely they are to suffer from mental health problems, drawing together unemployed factory workers of the Rust Belt, disaffiliated farmers of the Midwest, starving artists in California and Cuban migrants in Florida – to give a few sociologically based clichés. What does it mean, then, to be more likely to suffer from depression at the lower end of social hierarchy? To what extent can some contingent realities be merged in the same measurements or conceptualizations? What is the explanatory power of these correlations?

The problem is that thinking with variables often results in decontextualizing these realities. Most 'variables' are the product of particular contexts, and in a considerable number of cases, this context is the US. Take 'race'. In the US, 'race' has been institutionalized through colonization and slavery, before growing into a common set of idioms used to qualify people. In contrast, in France, it is deemed inappropriate to refer to someone's 'race' and racial statistics are prohibited (Fassin, 2011a). In the UK, partly out of sensitivities about colonialism and racism, suicide statistics have not historically reported on race/ethnicity; and it was only in recent decades that race/ethnic group was recorded on death certificates (Yue, 2021). In the countries of the former Yugoslavia, most 'Croatians', 'Bosnians', and 'Serbians' are white; however, administrative forms require individuals to state their 'ethnicity'. These meanings are *tied to history* (Wolfe, 2016) and this applies within the same country – compare Mississippi to Hawaii, or metropolitan and overseas France. What does it mean, then, to draw research findings on the relation between 'race' and mental health?[7] What does it mean to translate questionnaires with items dedicated to 'ethnicity' to be passed in several geographical areas? What can we exactly explain with the subsequent findings? These doubts, barely discussed in the literature, could be adapted to any variable presented above.

Last but not least, what do we really learn with correlations? Are we surprised that it is detrimental to live in poverty, to be alone, to be regularly discriminated against or to reside in unsafe neighbourhoods? Or that people living with the imminent fear of losing their job or being threatened due to their sexual orientation are more prone to depression or suicide? More accurately, that there is a social gradient in mental health? To be sure, some curiosity-inducing results have been enunciated, such as the 'epidemiological paradoxes' among migrants and African Americans, or the difficulty in identifying clear correlations in the case of social mobility. All of these findings are of the utmost significance, as they evidence a deep relation between mental illness and social stratifications; but at the same time, they are often relationships that might be expected. What, then, is the purpose of multiplying large-scale surveys, refining correlations, and developing more and more complex statistical tools, except – still crucially – to monitor and update the state of mental health inequalities? In other terms, now that we possess significant knowledge regarding the correlations tying mental health and social position, as well as the limitations of its measurements, and that several explanatory models have been generated, what is the future of this line of research?

To be clear, we do not mean that studies establishing correlation between indicators of mental health and of social position are irrelevant: they enlighten our knowledge of how alterity and its contingent forms affect mental health. We mean that these variable-based reasonings should be more systematically contextualized and that there are no self-sufficient findings: these should *only be a starting point* to understanding how social positions produce mental illness.

Beyond correlations: three alternatives

Once a path-breaking approach, the correlation paradigm has perhaps run its course. Correlating (decontextualized indicators of) mental health with (decontextualized indicators of) social position, in addition to relying on assumptions that are far from self-evident, as we have seen, is not enough to substantiate the 'pathogenic' effect of certain social locations. This realization, since the late twentieth century, paved the way for alternative perspectives that revolve around the *entanglement* of mental health and social position. Indeed, whereas for a correlation to be validly demonstrated, the correlating 'variables' must be relatively autonomous – mental health on one side, social position on the other – in our cases these variables are embedded, inter-related, inseparable. Social positions involve material and emotional dynamics *de facto* generating mental health states, and *simultaneously*, mental health issues emerge in certain contexts, with certain meanings, as fully-fledged parts of these sociocultural ecologies.

Remember Madame Bovary: her troubles cannot be isolated from the specific adversities of her objective social position (a women of the French rural bourgeoisie) and subjective positioning (her attraction to higher spheres), while the medical system is well prepared to pathologize any woman unhappy staying home waiting for their husband. Her 'nerve problems' are not *correlated with* gender and class; they are *part of* it. Madame Bovary's mental health and social position are co-occurring realities.

This section introduces three overlapping alternatives to the correlation paradigm: the *intersectional*, *configurational* and *definitional* perspectives.[8]

Intersectional perspectives

How might we embrace the complexity of social position and its role in producing and shaping mental health? The variables we discussed earlier have been extensively assessed one by one, and a current challenge therefore lies in understanding how they inter-relate. Do advantages and disadvantages amplify or neutralize one another, and how?

Intersectional perspectives offer a powerful resource to deal with these questions. They reconceptualize social position not as an addition of combined or independent aspects, instead addressing the interactions of these aspects in terms of meanings and effects, with a keen focus on power. Bowleg (2008, p 312) puts it well: 'Black + Lesbian + Woman ≠ Black Lesbian Woman.' This means that we cannot solely consider social characteristics as accumulating, as if we were adding comparable sums, for instance stacking age and gender within a regression analysis, or suggesting that black people have disadvantages that are 'worse' when combined with being a woman or being gay. Rather, intersectionality highlights the uniqueness and contingent nature of what makes social positions *intersectional* (Bowleg and Bauer, 2016). Arising as a theoretical construct from black feminist scholars, the concept was originally designed to theorize forms of domination such as violence against women (Crenshaw, 1991). Since its emergence, it has become a field of study, an analytical strategy and a critical praxis (Collins, 2015).

The intersectional framework has generated some impact in quantitative research, enabling questions to be posed regarding the 'tyranny of averages' (Evans and Erickson, 2019, p 3). However, the concept has been most widely taken up by qualitative researchers to examine how the social position of participants, in specific contexts, are embedded into structural forms of domination and inequality. If 'Black + Lesbian + Woman ≠ Black Lesbian Woman', then interviewing black lesbian women does not only entail studying femininity, blackness and homosexuality as layers of inequality. Rather, these 'variables' intertwine in a special fashion – and ultimately may not be understandable as variables at all.

However, the originality of these contributions often lack clarity: let us play devil's advocate for a paragraph. In quantitative research, intersectional models claim to differentiate themselves from 'classical' models because instead of listing dependent and independent variables and measuring their respective correlations, they introduce new statistical tools to capture the interaction between these variables (Seng et al, 2012; Villatoro et al, 2018a);[9] but this challenge preoccupied statisticians before intersectionality, and does not essentially transform quantitative operationalizations of social position in relation to mental health. In qualitative research, the trend to mobilize intersectionality in the cases of accumulating disadvantages (such as 'Black sexual minority men', English et al, 2020) obscures the benefit of this approach. Was it not already obvious, from the first urban ethnographies to traditional surveys on social stratification, that disadvantages combine and make up identities? As Carde (2021) points out, the main benefit of intersectionality lies in its potential to understand 'dissonant combinations', that is, individuals whose social position includes advantageous and disadvantageous attributes (such as gay men or wealthy black women).

Minimally, the intersectionality framework has served as an incentive to broaden the scope of social position in mental health research. It is through intersectionality that Mora-Rios et al (2016) enlarged their study on gender and the experience of schizophrenia in Mexico City to further incorporate dimensions of this experience such as caregiving duties and income in the family. Similarly, Viruell-Fuentes et al (2012) criticize the reduction of migrants' health to their 'culture', pointing to the impact of immigration policies and everyday discrimination articulated with gender and class on health – importantly highlighting the contextual meaning of these aspects (p 2104). And, when Kaiser, Näckter and Karlsson (2015) examine the situation of young Sami reindeer-herding females in Sweden – four 'variables' – they show how this singular social position arouses an ambivalence between pride related to Sami culture and the prestige of reindeer-herding, along with discrimination in relation to gender and ethnicity, contributing to mental ill-health, including suicidal thoughts. A key insight, again, is that beyond accumulated 'variables', intersectionality encourages the consideration of heterogeneous structural conditions, power and meaning.

Indeed, throughout these works, it appears that realizing the intersectional agenda requires paying particular attention to the meaning attached to social positioning. Sami herders do not only find themselves at the convergence of their gender, ethnicity, occupation and age: the meanings attributed to each of these attributes permeate their material conditions, experience and, ultimately, their mental health. This is how their social position manifests itself in their lives. For this reason, intersectional perspectives have contributed to remind sociologists of the importance of cultural representations attached to social hierarchies; this was already a classical sociological insight, at least since Weber, albeit often forgotten in mental health research, for instance in many studies focused on correlations. Donovan and West (2014) followed this path when they examine how 92 black women in the US relate to the stereotype of the 'strong black women', showing that endorsing this image can – perversely – render these women more vulnerable to stress, and distress. Collins et al's 2008 study of Latino women in New York in relation to mental illness and HIV integrates stereotypical figures of femininity as unique cultural references, that form a representational landscape in which mental distress is interpreted and makes sense. In sum, and *this should prevail beyond intersectional studies*, position and its meaning, and the embodied dynamics of social status, constitute an essential component of the social production of mental health.

An example of how these meanings are socially produced relates to how each disorder is situated in specific 'intersections', as in Widger's (2012) study on suicide in Madampe, Sri Lanka.[10] Three types of suicide are conceived by Sri Lankan people: *dukkha*, suicides of 'suffering', typically performed by middle class men; *asahanaya*, 'frustration' suicides for working class men; and *kopeya*, suicides of 'anger', for working class women. Thus,

> Suicidal performances and their accompanying discourses become literal and figurative battlegrounds upon which local class and gender ideologies and structures are affirmed or denied, in some cases asserting notions of masculinity and middle-class power and control and in others maintaining or challenging subordinate female roles and

working class prejudice. In turn, class, and gender concerns shape individuals' pathways to suicidal acts, shaping why, how, and with what consequences they may be performed. (Widger, 2012, p 226)

In its most extensive form, such attention to meanings can be derived in 'critical phenomenology'. Close to Ahmed's 'queer phenomenology' (2006), this approach puts the effect of inequalities and structural patterns of domination in perspective within the very construction of meanings at stake in mental health-related problems. Chandler's (2019) work on suicide illustrates this approach. She notes that, when reflecting on their self-harming behaviours and suicidal distress, white working class men in the UK express embodied distress and difficulty in facing their 'failures' and the feeling of 'being stopped', as their position (socially and historically) comes with the expectation of neat and stable trajectories (job, family, prestige) which – because of structural factors – they had not seen realized. In such cases, thoughts of suicide, or acts of self-harm, were reframed as a positive action – a body that could still do at least one thing. Critical phenomenology, in reconciling phenomenology with its Marxist critique (that phenomenology would be blind to social divides), thus points to the substantial contributions that an intersectional perspective can have in mental health research, incorporating meaning and experience to understand *how* intersecting social positions may produce mental ill-health and related outcomes.

In sum, intersectional perspectives have impelled significant transformations in how sociology can approach inequalities in relation to mental health. More than a set of variables, inequalities were reframed as intersections between various hierarchies, and, close to the classical distinction established by Bourdieu (1979, 1980) between objective and subjective position, we have suggested that a fertile area of investigation lies in the (not necessarily new) interface between social stratifications and the meaning attached to these.

From this perspective, mental disorders are embedded in the inter-relations between someone's position among multiple social hierarchies that structure their social environment and the meanings they can attribute to their place in this context.

Configurational perspectives

While intersectional perspectives construct mental health as the emanation of how gender, class, age and so on entangle in a unique way *within* individuals (for instance, Milan is a white middle class 50 year old man residing in a wealthy district in Hungary), configurational approaches further accentuate the components that construct social positions *around* the individuals (so, in addition, Milan grew up in a working class family, his wife comes from the British aristocracy and he socializes with many people of colour at work).

The difference is slight, and porous, but we still make this distinction to emphasize the span of reasonings to be possibly examined. Another way of explaining this difference is that while the notion of intersectionality emphasizes the multiple properties that make up people's social position, the notion of configuration[11] encompasses the properties not only of the groups an individual might belongs to, but also those with which they interact. There are several ways to conceptualize this approach, from the work of Weber, who defends a 'multi-integrative ethnography' (Weber, 2001) later applied to 'care configurations' and kinship around people suffering from mental disorders (Blum et al, 2015; Béliard et al, 2018), to Price-Robertson et al's (2017) more theoretical proposal to approach mental health and recovery through 'family assemblage' taken as an 'assemblage of heterogeneous components (e.g. bodies, practices, objects, stories and everyday interactions)' (p 413). Several overlapping reasonings can be drawn from this standpoint.

Some studies focus on *specific groups*, or *classes*, and understand their emotion and mental health through the prism of their relation to other groups or classes. Two studies of anxiety provide useful illustrations. Fong (2011) relates the pressures experienced by Chinese-born elite international students, explored in relation to the investment they are made the object of in families restricted by the one-child policy. Sherman (2017) interviews affluent New Yorkers and witnesses a singular type of anxiety, the 'anxiety of affluence'. Her participants developed a justificatory narrative of their wealth that largely depends on their milieu of origin (whether they inherited or not) and who they are acquainted with (whether they compare themselves with richer or 'poorer' people). Both Fong and Sherman portray forms of anxiety that are entrenched into unique configurations, made not only of how people internalize their social position (as per the intersectional perspective) but how the studied groups (Chinese students and rich New Yorkers) situate themselves objectively and subjectively in relation to other groups (Chinese parents and different fractions of the US upper classes) which itself depends on historically constructed, local social stratification systems (the one-child policy in China, increasing global and national inequalities).

Some social positions seem to be, in themselves, *productive of distress*. Scheper-Hughes (1977), in her ethnography of rural Ireland, noted that people diagnosed with schizophrenia were often the second sons of families whose farm was in economic crisis, but who were still morally 'condemned' to take it over while their older brothers and any daughters could migrate to cities and, there, benefit from more life opportunities. In her study of primary school teachers in France, Balland (2020) analyses these teachers' anxiety as an 'unfortunate and socially situated relationship to a position' (p 83), that is, a tension between the institutional constraints affecting their work and their aspirations drenched in idealism. In all these cases, distress, and eventually mental health issues, are parts of the processes by which people try to adjust to the composite configuration in which they live.

Configurational perspectives can contribute to making sense of otherwise contradictory findings of some statistical studies, which (perhaps surprisingly) do not establish a correlation between *social mobility and mental disorders*. Such approaches underline the importance of the different meanings which social mobility takes on in different contexts and situations. Does the experience of mobility leave, as Friedman (2015) theorizes in Britain, an 'emotional imprint' through the creation of a 'cleft habitus' within the same person? Back in the 1980s, in France, De Gaulejac (1987) created a concept to describe the 'main characteristics of psychological conflicts related to social status' and social mobility (p 15): 'class neurosis'. The 'clinical picture' of class neurosis includes feelings of 'guilt and inferiority', 'of being divided from the inside', 'particular difficulties in facing the Oedipus complex' and 'isolation and withdrawal' (p 150). The adversity of social mobility has been observed in many settings, such as among people experiencing upward mobility from the British working class (Hoggart, 1957, 238–259) or among students. Cant (2017) studied distress among students in the UK through the notion of hysteresis: suggesting this was produced by a lack of fit between the expectations of their current environment and those they had been socialized to.

A relatively untapped way to further examine this issue consists of identifying precise *moments pivotal to social trajectories*. Thus Allouch's (2021) work on the selection committees for French elite universities approaches oral examinations as rituals where students are expected to produce two types of emotion work: on the one hand, displaying 'mandatory anxiety' to convey their concern for the examination, deemed a normal outcome of competition; and, on the other hand, showing that they can overcome their anxiety for the sake of intellectual performance. In sum, certain aspects of social mobility, in certain configurations, generate emotions and life conditions that relate more or less directly to mental health.

The *strategies by which people achieve social mobility or try to 'find their place'* opens another outlook to this question. Much research shows how individuals from disadvantaged backgrounds engage in sustained efforts to palliate the negative stereotypes they fear their interlocutors imagine, but that this comes with a 'psychological' cost, as in the US for black professional women managing discrimination (Bacchus, 2008) or people speaking with an accent (Lippi-Green, 2012).

In other cases, *strategies of social positioning are themselves the symptoms*. For instance, Darmon's (2017) work on anorexia in France draws on interviews with young women diagnosed with anorexia. Darmon argues that anorexia embodies a lifestyle change aimed at moving closer to the ethos of the upper classes. Indeed, since anorexia not only encompasses a reduction in the quantity of food consumed, but also a qualitative change in how food is consumed, and incorporated into an 'ascetic' lifestyle – eating less to read and study more. The social practices of anorectic young women, according to Darmon, attempt to replicate the (projected) lifestyle of those at the top of the social hierarchy prizing thinness, spending time learning 'legitimate culture'. This work resonates with that of Katzman et al (2004), who found that all identified cases of anorexia in Curaçao (in the Caribbean) were 'mixed race', relatively affluent young women with more access to international travel and educational opportunities than the majority black population of the island. In these works, mental disorders are not only the 'psychological costs' of mobility but entangle with the various practices that make social positioning, and eventually mobility, possible in the first place.

As the study of configurations decentres social inquiry from the troubled individual to consider the various groups in which they live, it can lead to identify *socially produced, recurrent relational dynamics*. Brossard's (2018) study of self-injury in Francophone countries raises attention to the family, residential and school configurations in which those who self-injure find themselves. Often characterized by tensions surrounding social mobility, gender and class display, these configurations can be studied in asking about the social positions of each family member and how this affects their relations – for instance parents from different social backgrounds, conflicts between different factions of the family, or residential situations creating a feeling of discrepancy with the neighbourhood. Another example is provided by Pearson and Liu (2002), who concentrate on the case of a woman who died by suicide in rural China. They show that the social environment of this suicide is not only a combination of factors, but also a story where family relations, religion, integration in a local community, income, gendered expectations and customs (the family of the wronged daughter who died by suicide could destroy their in-laws possessions) mingle.[12] Mental disorders 'make sense in' configurations.

In sum, configurational perspectives approach mental health problems as the reflection of issues that affect the social configurations in which people live, which can include unfortunate positions, social mobilities, strategies of social positioning and more specific configurational dynamics.

Definitional perspectives

Definitional perspectives suggest that the link between mental health and social position cannot be unproblematically examined as a correlation, because the very definition and management of mental disorders in societies *reflects and contributes to the construction of social divides*. Not only do mental health categories often target certain publics and convey socially situated norms, but they also partly produce these publics and participate in naturalizing their stratification. This idea can be broken down into three reasonings: 1) professionals use categories and related practices that reflect their own – situated – worldview; 2) mental health categories are, therefore, socially situated ideals; 3) the way that mental disorders are defined leads to certain groups being targeted, relating to particular life conditions, or to situated emotional practices. We discuss each of these in turn.

Firstly, *professionals use categories and practices that often echo their own, situated, representation of the world*. In the 1950s, Hollingshead and Redlich (1958) had noted that working class psychiatric patients were hospitalized for longer periods of time and were less likely to receive talking therapies than upper class patients. Doctors perhaps thought that such patients would be less receptive to talking – indeed, they did not talk in the same way as the doctors themselves. More recently, Holman (2014) used qualitative interviews, and a Bourdieusian theoretical framework, to attempt to explain why in the UK working class patients – despite higher rates of diagnosed depression and anxiety – were referred less often for talking therapies than middle class patients. He argued that talking therapies require socially situated – middle class coded – dispositions to be effective, that is, inclinations towards 'verbalisation and introspection, impetus for emotional health, relation to medical authority and practical orientation to the future' (p 542); such configurations of therapy can exclude, explicitly or implicitly, working class patients.

Other works show that mental health professionals' actions and assumptions in relation to patients both draws on and reinforces social positions (their own and their patients'). Ethnographies of psychiatric wards could demonstrate with both class – see Coutant and Eideliman (2013) on how French psychiatry was used to 'govern by listening' the adolescent working class, with ambivalent effects on the patients' social trajectories – and gender – psychiatry reinforces gender expectations in various ways (see Feyeux, 2021, in France or Pinto, 2014, in India). More historical approaches and discourse analysis show significant gendered expectations in psychiatry (Ussher, 2011; Haggett, 2015; Busfield, 2017). In a nutshell, and as a consequence, the mental health apparatus 'acts on' social stratification.

Mainly focusing on the US, Hirshbein (2009) demonstrates that depression emerged in the nineteenth century on the basis of deeply gendered assumptions, rephrased as biological differences between men and women. Psychiatrists, men, wanted to help these women, already deemed more fragile and vulnerable to their emotions, who developed 'irrationally' high expectations regarding domestic happiness and, disappointed, experienced intense phases of sadness (think back to Emma Bovary). This representation stabilized over the twentieth century through a circular process: 'women were believed to be depressed more than men and were selected for clinical trials more than men, and then their greater presence within trials appeared to affirm that they were depressed more than men' (Hirshbein, 2009, p 90). Diagnostic criteria were constructed out of these gendered representations, that is, the *definition* of depression was gendered from the outset, originally tailored to fit the troubles of women – as seen by men – generating its own epidemiological, circular reality; which contributes to explain the correlation between depression and gender in statistical surveys. A similar argument is seen in relation to the gendering of self-injury in Chandler et al (2011). In contrast, other disorders have been constructed as more masculine, and clinical trials included more men, such as autism (Baron-Cohen, 2002).

As such, the social composition of the professionals in charge of defining mental disorders affects how mental health issues are socially defined, and thus how a mental health framework is used more to understand the issues of certain publics – in the case of depression, psychiatrists labelling women. Decades of research, treatments and medical socialization then reproduce the status quo, offering further legitimacy to gender, but also class, age and race related differences.

The social position of mental health professionals has a direct repercussion on the definition of mental disorders and how they target, if not construct, certain populations. This process, despite the wealth of research conducted on professions, remains underexplored. What is the effect of the relative feminization of mental health professions over the twentieth century (Adams, 2010; Kirkpatrick, 2004)? What is the effect of the rise of psychology and personal development, as they correspond to serious professional changes in the mode of selection and training of these occupations? Although we have prioritized class and gender in our discussion here, the same reasoning applies to any aspect of social position such as age, since mental health professionals are adults working with certain representations of childhood, adolescence and ageing, or race.[13]

The second reasoning we identify is that *mental health categories express socially situated ideals* – reflecting the values of those generating and using particular definitions of mental disorder. In this reasoning, the norms expressed through psychiatric (and psychological) categories are not 'neutral' but promote political worldviews on social order attached to the interests and worldviews of certain groups.

From this perspective, taking mental health categories and reversing them is an instructive exercise for sociologists which illustrates this well: in doing so, we can excavate the crude contours of what is understood to be 'normal' in a given society, at a given time. Cohen (2016) provides a cogent example. Listing DSM symptoms, he reflects on the contemporary definition of mental health, which mainly designates situations where people are not effective at work, at school, or eventually with their family. Someone's inability to focus (disturbed by ADHD and addictions), to feel stable emotions (disturbed by bipolar disorder or borderline personality disorder), to stay 'sociable' (disturbed by depression, social anxiety, certain forms of schizophrenia) and to restrict one's eccentricity to reasonable limits (disturbed by autism) troubles the pillars of traditional social functioning – a social order for the middle and upper classes. Examining the successive versions of DSM, Cohen observes that despite the feminization of the labour force, the classification manual increasingly promotes traditional feminine roles, through sex-role clichés of women taken primarily as wives, mothers, carers and home makers, from dedicating specific categories to women, such as the Premenstrual Dysphoric Disorder (pp 152–153), to 'replacing' the traditionally feminized hysteria with borderline personality disorder (pp 156–164). He also observes an increase in categories pathologizing young people (p 114), among other fractions of the population. Cohen concludes that the conservative, dominant and omnipresent aspect of the mental health apparatus today represents a *psychiatric hegemony*.

Some research uses critical discourse analysis to deconstruct the latent meanings of mental health categories in view of their economic, social, cultural and political contexts. From a cultural studies perspective, Jaworski (2010) criticizes the Western representation of suicide as an individual, deliberate act that can be either 'achieved' or 'missed', which presumes a masculinist cultural understanding of 'success' and 'completion' and by extension, frames ('feminine') self-harm as a 'failure'. River and Flood (2021) show how such meaning is endorsed by Australian men as an alternative means of demonstrating masculinity, whereby the body became both the vehicle and object of violence. From a policy analysis perspective, Braedley (2012) argues that Ontario health care policy (as most Western policies), while claiming to follow a 'neutral' logic combining neoliberal tenets and the medical paradigm, ultimately promotes 'elite masculine norms' such as instrumental rationality, objectivity, calculation and control over dependent persons. In a wide review, which includes policy analysis, Prior (1999, p 77) summarizes that 'definitions of normality are almost always tied to gendered notions of behaviour and ways of thinking'; here again, we could add class, age, and so forth.

The third, and final, reasoning identified in relation to definitional perspectives on the stratification of mental health, observes and interrogates how *mental disorders are defined in ways which lead to certain groups being targeted*. This plays out in two ways: the definitions of some mental disorders correspond closely to the life conditions of particular groups (we relate this to trauma, and to surveillance); and in other cases, the criteria for diagnoses resonate with the emotional specialization of particular groups.

Tseris (2019) shows that the emergence of trauma as a core concept for psy-professionals around the world raised hopes of empowering women, by acknowledging types of violence that particularly affect them. The creation of this way of making sense of and categorizing mental illness thus relates to the existence of violent oppression, which tends to target particular groups (women, racialized ethnic groups, LGBT+ people). However, Tseris argues that current theoretical and practical elaborations likely generate the opposite effect: today, the 'trauma paradigm' tends to erase a diversity of experiences into one model, to focus on a neuro-biochemical level of understanding that individualizes troubles and, thereby, shifts the attention to the individual *consequences* of traumatic events rather than their social *cause*. As a result, this conception can divert or minimize attempts towards social change, instead naturalizing the psychologization of women's experiences, and overlooking the structural reasons why women experience gender-based violence.

Harper (2011) starts from the premise that individuals, depending on their gender, class and race, have different experiences of surveillance, safety and control. In the UK and elsewhere, people of colour are more likely to suffer from discrimination and being more 'watched'. Women are less safe in public spaces, more observed. Working class people are subject to more control by the state, they are more suspected of fraud, especially when unemployed. As a consequence, paranoia is not only embedded in these experiences but sometimes justified, so to speak. While, Harper theorizes, the DSM includes some mentions that a delusional state is characterized by its non-acceptance in the culture or subculture of the person, these mentions are vague and probably not always thought as such by psychiatrists interacting with women, people of colour or those who are working class. Asking whether psychiatrists individually might recognize the role of socially stratified experiences for particular patients is not the point: as we will elaborate in the next chapter, at a social level, paranoia cannot be understood individually without examining more widely the unequal context in which trust can be formulated and experienced. Here again, a symptomatology deemed socially neutral – delusional paranoia – appears to be, in practice, inseparable from the social stratifications in which the position of the concerned persons takes place and makes sense.

A related, but distinct, way in which mental disorders can be seen to target particular groups, addresses diversity in emotional expression, experience and meaning. In line with the 'artefact explanation' mentioned earlier, some works, either because they study specific milieux or because they analyse specific diagnostic tools, have the potential to question current knowledge on prevalence rates of many disorders. Alang (2016) suggests that African American people in the US express distress in ways that are less detected by usual psychiatric assessment, since they consider, more than white people, depression as a sign of weakness to be dismissed or rephrased – or that it is not a real illness – and use other words, metaphors and emotional manifestations to express sadness. Similarly, Hirshbein (2009) criticizes the Center for Epidemiologic Studies Depression Scale (CES-D), probably the most widely used questionnaire in mental health studies worldwide, for half of its questions centring on expressions of self-feeling, that women are more likely to answer. Thus, the common finding that rates of depression are lower among African American people, and higher among women may relate to the way that the criteria for these disorders are constructed – what constitutes depression is implicitly coded to align with emotional styles among particular groups.

Cheslack-Postava and Jordan-Young (2012) theorize this perspective further, attending to both biological and social dimensions of mental health. Trying to explain why more men are diagnosed with autism than women, they propose an 'embodiment model'. Starting with the idea that 'biologically based vulnerabilities', such as those related to sensory and cognitive abilities, exist and may be sex-linked, they argue that gender socialization may shape how far, and whether, these vulnerabilities manifest into behaviours associated with autism. They draw on existing studies that show how mundane behaviours that are central in the diagnosis of autism – such as making eye-contact and the recognition of emotions in interaction – dramatically differ between boys and girls due to how boys and girls are raised from early childhood. They suggest then that autism symptoms are embedded within male emotional socialization, leading men to be more likely to develop behavioural patterns associated with autism and, thus, to be more widely diagnosed.

Conclusion

Social position and mental health do not only correlate: they are entangled. In this chapter, our main argument has been that the turn taken by much mental health research since the 1980s regarding the 'relation' between mental disorder 'and' social position somehow lost its way, privileging technical details over reflecting on *how* this relation operates. Variables are relational, in the sense that they make sense only in context and need to be historicized so they can be used in explanatory argumentations.

Thus, we reorganized contemporary literature into three alternative approaches (intersectional, configurational and definitional) that hold the potential to overcome this problem. These alternatives, though, raise further questions: for instance, what does mental health *do* to social stratification, and vice versa? Does the mental health apparatus act as a conservative force trying to entrench traditional social divides, or a 'reifier' of the social structure naturalizing the values of certain groups, or sometimes as an accelerator of social change? Deeper investigations into this co-productive link between mental illness and social divides would make all the more sense as historically, Western psychiatry emerged along with the transition from a paternalistic social order to a class-based society (Scull, 1989).

A final point should be raised as an opening: we cannot continue without posing the problem of social justice. In most of the perspectives we discuss lurks the denunciation of the 'side effects' of social inequalities. Many researchers critique deprivation, discrimination, structural racism and sexism as producers of mental distress. Others identify at-risk communities, or risk factors, to account for the specific 'needs' of these vulnerable populations, such as queer people, migrants or disadvantaged neighbourhoods. Access to care is another source of inequality. Most of these works point to the impossibility of distinguishing mental health inequalities from the wider inequalities in which they take place. However, arguably, in our societies where labour is supposed to be motivational, because the wealth it sometimes provides supposedly increases wellbeing, these general inequalities are not a dysfunction, fixable by a few mental health policies; they are a *functional basis* for capitalist economies to thrive. Social and economic inequalities might therefore, *quite logically, without surprise and even intentionally*,[14] generate inequalities in mental health. As such, can we criticize mental health inequalities as unfair differences in the experiences of social life, without simultaneously criticizing economic inequalities and cultural distinctions at large? Returning to Madame Bovary: should we help her to more happily inhabit her social position, or reduce the inequalities of the society she lives in? Perhaps both of these? From this standpoint, and this is rarely discussed in the reviewed literature, researching mental health inequalities, very fundamentally, engages a political philosophy of what inequalities mean for social organization.

2

Society as Stressor

Anyone familiar with the world of mental health would read *Veronika Decides to Die* (Coelho, 1998) with some surprise. Veronika, a young woman from Slovenia, whose life appears to be otherwise 'good', tries to kill herself. When she wakes up, her psychiatrist tells her that the medicine she took triggered a toxic reaction that has only postponed her death. She will pass away in a few weeks. During these weeks, Veronika reflects on her situation, meets some patients from her ward, falls in love with one of them, and, ultimately, learns to appreciate life. The twist of this story is unveiled at the end. Her psychiatrist admits that he lied. Veronika will live.

In many respects, this novel runs counter to psychiatric common sense. Firstly, what motivates Veronika's suicide attempt is not adversity, distress or trauma, but the meaninglessness of her trouble-free existence – a *lack* of stress. That said, it is through pressuring Veronika into an irreversible death sentence that her psychiatrist provides the much-needed shock that would give meaning to her life and spark some vital energy.

This story offers a counter-narrative to a major trend in the sociology of mental health: the *stress paradigm*. The stress paradigm incorporates a vast range of works that study how various difficulties, from discrimination to car accidents through sexual abuse and other traumas, generate stress; and how stress, when not buffered with the appropriate, material and 'psychological' resources, is a catalyst for mental disorders.

One of the oldest explanations in the history of ideas seeking to make sense of 'madness', though phrased initially as pressure or overburdening, stress was introduced to sociology through biology. Armed with this multiform concept, quantitative sociologists were able to measure various pathways towards mental distress. The set of factors they identified enabled collaborations with psychology and psychiatry, facilitating the integration of social factors into mainstream interpretations of mental health. However, although the stress paradigm provided some ground on which to imagine how social factors generate individual troubles through unequal exposure to adversity, some major gaps tarnish its explanatory power. Most pressingly, 'stress' is an umbrella term used to compare and contrast widely different situations; in doing so, it reduces the nuances of human emotions at play in the social genesis of mental disorders, not least their embodied, emotional, unequal and culturally diverse expressions (Busfield, 1996).

Starting with the seminal works of Hans Selye (1956), this chapter reviews the current state of play in this area, emphasizing that the most dominant sociological model of stress – Pearlin's 'stress process model' – is embedded into longer term thinking about the effects of modern, urban life, and that its biological underpinning originally conveys hope to overcome the mind/body divide. But the lure of biologically based models of stress has enrolled sociological thinking in increasingly reductionist directions. Many current uses of stress lack sociological imagination, individualizing reactions to stress, referring to social contexts as quite abstract entities, and universalizing stress, hermetic to repeated studies that demonstrate the cultural and historical variations of its meaning (Jackson, 2013, Bendelow, 2009).

This chapter proposes two productive avenues that build on the rich body of work generated by those inspired by the stress paradigm, but which move beyond some of the limitations we identify. Firstly, we advance that studies of stress need to systematically situate stress within the power relations that generate its onset, intensity, meaning and consequences. With this reflection already initiated in feminist approaches and the concept of 'minority stress' (Meyer, 2003), we need to consider the long histories and continuing enactments of oppression that frame types of stress within broader economic structures, among others, as in Mark Fisher's (2011) meditations on the 'privatization of stress' and its relationship to capitalism. Critically considering the effects of contemporary sociological imaginings of stress (Thomas et al, 2020), we secondly call for a fuller engagement with the sociological nature of emotions (Schieman, 2019), and examine some possibilities to 'sociologize' the generative power of emotions beyond the generic notion of stress. Considering these approaches illuminates the limitations of more functionalist, conservative sociological imaginations which inflect much research on stress, mental disorder and emotions (Cobb, 2018).

Rise and decline of the stress paradigm

This first section provides an overview of the historical origins of the concept of stress, and the development of the stress paradigm. We chart some of the key insights generated by stress researchers regarding the social genesis of mental disorders. This includes the ways in which stress research allows for engagement with the entangled nature of sociological and biological understandings of mental health. Finally, we examine some key limitations of the stress paradigm: its problematic assumptions regarding the universality and measurability of stress; its abstraction of 'context'; its underlying moral conservatism; and lastly, its ineffectiveness in generating novel findings.

Social origins: stress in the city

Put charitably, stress is a 'flexible' concept, literally denoting a pressure being applied to someone, the image of a weight, worry or tension. It evokes the disturbance of a state of equilibrium (stress *versus* health and wellbeing), and thus its origins can be traced as far back as Hippocratic and Galenic medicine, and early ideas of homeostasis and health (Jackson, 2013). From the late nineteenth into the twentieth centuries, discussion of stress among scientists and within popular culture[1] was widespread and changed in tenor: stress became an object of science first and later a market – consider the wide array of industries that promise to reduce the stress of their customers today (Jackson, 2013; Roberts and McWade, 2021). Such concerns with emotional stability were echoed among social scientists writing in the early twentieth century, with a focus on the alleged challenges of rapid social change. This is epitomized in Georg Simmel's (2010) meditations on the psychic impacts of increasing urbanization, which he framed around the development of a 'blasé outlook' – understood as a psychic defence to the potentially overwhelming nature of city life:

> There is perhaps no psychic phenomenon which is so unconditionally reserved to the city as the blasé outlook ... Just as an immoderately sensuous life makes one blasé because it stimulates the nerves to their utmost reactivity until they finally can no longer produce any reaction at all, so, less harmful stimuli, through the rapidity, and the contradictoriness of their shifts, force the nerves to make such violent responses, tear them about so brutally that they exhaust their last reserves of strength. (Simmel, 2010, p 14)

Studies of the city and mental life provide a useful illustration of how sociology has sought to imagine how the communities, geographies, jobs and relationships that individuals inhabit may act as 'stressors' or 'buffers'. Current understandings of stress build on links drawn between 'modernity' and wellbeing, the psychological impacts of busy, highly populated, highly stratified city life, rooted in older notions of health, self and social order. Early studies of mental disorder within cities raised (enduring) concerns that city life is 'bad' for mental health, leading to higher rates of depression, anxiety and – especially – psychosis (Fitzgerald et al, 2016a, 2016b). This latter consideration is especially of interest, since psychosis is often framed as different from other disorders among many sociologies of mental health, viewed as more likely to be biologically rather than socially driven (Metzl,

2010). Despite this, a major finding of studies across the twentieth and twenty-first century is a strong correlation between living, or being born, in a city and later development of psychotic symptoms, or a psychosis diagnosis (Fitzgerald et al, 2016a; Li and Liu, 2018).

The city has been a key research focus for sociologists in general. The activities centring around the Chicago School of sociology, and the city as a 'living lab' in the formation of a still emergent discipline is an oft cited example (Fitzgerald et al, 2016b). Equally important, and increasingly recognized, is the work of W.E.B. Du Bois in Philadelphia (Du Bois, 2007; Bhambra, 2014). Each of these focal points generated studies of cities as geographical, social, cultural sites through which to explore the shaping of human experiences and trajectories, to understand the social patterning of life – and associated health inequalities. Early ecological studies of cities sought to develop fine-grained and geographically sensitive accounts of how place of dwelling related to rates of different forms of mental disorder. But the study of urban communities did not lead to a systematic approach to stress. This was to come, initially, from biology.

From the origins of stress to the stress paradigm

In the twentieth century, Hans Selye (1956) popularized a version of stress which remains the most influential. Selye observed adaptive disorders in rats when faced with a range of 'shocks' from actual electric shocks to chemical 'shocks' via exposure to formaldehyde. His work demonstrated a relationship between structural changes to rat's brains, and functional changes in their behaviour, following such exposure (Youdell et al, 2018). He expanded these insights to humans, advancing a social philosophy of stress which drew on theories regarding the impacts of chronic stressors on hormonal functions, specifically adreno-cortical responses (Jackson, 2013, pp 112–113). Selye's original work seeded a whole range of further developments and tangents as subsequent research builds on his initial insights regarding a biological basis for human and non-human adaptation to stressors, many of them social in origin.

In sociology, a key originator of theories about the impact of stress on mental illness is Leonard Pearlin (Aneshensel and Avison, 2015; Pearlin, 1989). Pearlin's work converted the early historical concepts of stress into operational sociological methodology, via a focus on balance between individual resources and social stressors, an approach in which bodies and biology are notably absent. Pearlin (et al, 1981) first tested this approach with a longitudinal study of 1,106 people living in the Chicago area, based on standardized scales. He demonstrated correlations between variables deemed indicative of stress and psychological distress: the more we are stressed, the more we experience distress. Although the idea itself was not new, it was probably the first time that numbers substantiated this correlation. Ultimately, Pearlin's approach triggered the unification of works within the sociology of mental health around the representation of mental health issues as produced by and resulting in stress. Any problematic emotions associated with mental health issues, in this frame, can be converted into 'stress', that is, both a conceptual elaboration compatible with most theoretical perspectives, and methodologically operationalizable tools, quantitative and qualitative (Aneshensel and Avison, 2015).

This perspective indeed speaks to a number of concerns in our disciplines, such as linkages between social factors and mental health, the role of biology within this, as well as ways of accounting for the nature and multiplicity of social adversity, from situational difficulties to structural inequalities. In addition, the notion of 'stress' offers us a flexible metaphor (often steeped in mechanistic or engineering imaginaries) through which to understand *how* challenging life events, ongoing stressors, or long histories of trauma and oppression may produce disordered minds. Thus, the stress paradigm was applicable in different areas of research, such as the mental health of migrants (Noh and Avison, 1996), gender inequalities (Kessler and McLeod, 1984) and neighbourhood effects on mental illness (Stockdale et al, 2007). It has been dominant in Anglophone mental health sociology since the 1980s, especially in the US (Thoits, 1995; Schwartz, 2002). A key reason for this success may lie in this ability of stress models to articulate a methodologically explorable, causal relationship between social context and mental disorder.

We could summarize this paradigm as follows: a sustainable mismatch between challenging situations and an individual's resources to handle them constitutes the fundamental mechanism in the aetiology of mental disorders.

Identifying forms of stress, therefore, is of great significance for proponents of the stress paradigm, who generally distinguish between:

- stress originating from significant or traumatic life events (such as divorce, trauma);
- chronic stress leading from ongoing experiences (chronic illness, poverty or unemployment); and
- 'daily hassles', ranging from relatively mundane issues (like a 'car breakdown') to those related to social structure (such as racial microaggressions).[2]

But stress does not mechanically produce distress. This is why another area of exploration concerns how this relation operates and can be mediated: investigating the *buffer effect* played by social support and coping skills; *the impact of stress*, estimating what, in the stressful events themselves, determines their propensity to generate distress (Thoits, 1995; Pearlin, 1989); and *dispositions to handle stress*, or how individuals' trajectories prior to the stressor could explain its impact on their mental health (Wheaton, 1990). The success of the stress paradigm led to a multiplication of explanatory schemas (Ensel and Lin, 1991) where sources of stress, called 'stressors', resources to cope with them and emotional distress – this distress being considered as a premise for various mental illnesses – can be either causes, resources, buffers or outcomes.

Biological imaginaries of 'stressed minds'

Among other explanatory models of mental disorder, a singularity of the stress paradigm lies in its biological origin. The concept of stress relates closely to notions of biological equilibrium and balance because it does not exactly denote something stressful, or how people feel about being stressed, but rather points to stress as a bodily reaction *in* those subjects to stressful lives or stressful events. Medical research shows that stress, far from being solely 'mental', has multiple and durable ramifications in the body, from modifying hormones to activating parts of the brain, from modifying blood pressure to affecting the immune system (Roberts and McWade, 2021). As such, stress provides one route (among many) for potentially rethinking the Cartesian mind/body divide, whose influence is problematic for understanding mental health (Bendelow, 2009), yet which remains so pervasive in accounts and explanations of mental health.

The stress model inspired early interdisciplinary collaborations, mostly between sociologists and psychiatrists, showing evidence of a 'fleshy' or bodily understanding of stressed city dwellers (Fitzgerald et al, 2016b). However, this early flirtation with interdisciplinarity was largely abandoned over the latter half of the twentieth century, mirroring a similar shift away from collaborations with psychiatry (Pilgrim and Rogers, 2005). In recent years interdisciplinary partnerships have again opened up, with 'new' biosciences of genetics, epigenetics and stress hormones proving to be productive focuses for sociology to engage more deeply with the embodiment, and bodily traces of, social stress (Fitzgerald et al, 2016a; McEwen and McEwen, 2017; Mort et al, 2019; Youdell et al, 2018; Roberts and McWade, 2021).

In the realm of genetics, for instance Schnittker (2010), drawing on data from the University of Washington Twin Registry, argues that the relationship between stress and depression appears to be mediated at least partly by genes. Using the same database, Beam and colleagues (2017) examined how genes might slightly mediate a relationship between self-reported stress and marriage. Where researchers attempt to engage with social and biological drivers and mediators of both stress as outcome, and a relationship between stress and mental disorders, often surprising results ensue. For instance, Beam et al (2017) find that in contrast to the usual finding that stress increases more for women who are married than it does for men, when including genetic similarity or difference in statistical models, marriage appears to *reduce* perceived stress among women who might otherwise be genetically predisposed to report more stress. That said, findings are rarely equivocal, and gene-environment studies (and the twin studies on which they are often based) are still emergent, hugely complex and contested (Pickersgill et al, 2013; Joseph, 2013; Viney, 2016).

The biology of stress has been especially influenced by the development of measures of cortisol – the so-called 'stress hormone' (Roberts and McWade, 2021). Cortisol level measurements have been used as a proxy to follow how stress evolves throughout a day of work (Kunz-Ebrecht et al, 2004), or before and after an event such as visiting a cultural heritage site (Grossi et al, 2019). Such measurements were employed in the Northeast US by Damaske et al (2014) to argue that stress levels are higher at home than at work. With experimental methods, Taylor measured gender differences in responses to being a 'token male/female' in the workplace, and being socially excluded. She found that there was no biological difference (measured via cortisol) in responses to this scenario, arguing this underlined that differences in 'stress' among men and women were more likely to be attributable to social contexts rather than an 'essential' gender difference in the capacity to tolerate stress (Taylor, 2016). However, the assumption that cortisol levels amount to stress levels remains debatable.

US sociologist Craig McEwen and neuroendocrinologist Bruce McEwen, who has carried out pioneering work on the notion of 'allostatic load', have argued strongly for an agenda of interdisciplinary work where sociologists and scientists of the biology of stress can work together productively to better understand and intervene in the troubling relationships between social structure, poverty, adversity, 'toxic' stress and poor outcomes for children (McEwen and McEwen, 2017). The message is positive – and reflects some of the optimism discussed by Fitzgerald et al (2016a) regarding the productive possibilities of interdisciplinary collaborations between sociology and biology.

> Rather than weakening sociological explanations, the introduction of biological mechanisms relating to toxic stress strengthens these explanations by recognizing biological processes ... through which social inequalities become embodied, especially in the early childhood years. (McEwen and McEwen, 2017, p 447)

For sociologists of stress, McEwen and McEwen suggest that learning from biological or specifically neuroendocrinological insights can help to open up the 'black box' of correlations between social inequalities and health outcomes, especially where those inequalities and hardships are experienced among children. These proposals are compelling – and reflect much of the allure identified by critical commentaries on interdisciplinary engagements between sociology and neuroscience, and sociology and genetics (Callard and Fitzgerald, 2015; Pickersgill et al, 2013). These engagements take place in a history where sociologists have been suspicious of 'biological reductionism', and in stress research this has meant that in many cases the potential role of biological mechanisms are overlooked entirely. We do not wish to replicate overly pessimistic positions about the reductionism of biological explanations. However, we do want to highlight a number of significant cautions in how some of the literature on the sociology of stress has articulated these relationships, and the problems this may cause in our attempts to understand the relationship between society and mental disorder.

McEwen and McEwen's 2017 paper focuses especially on the impact of childhood adversity on children's educational outcomes and performance, reading this as a proxy for wellbeing in later life. There is a lot to unpick here regarding the assumptions that are made, and the focus of the interventions that the paper implies and proposes. For instance, drawing on Michelle Lareau's (2002) study of differing parental styles across working class and middle class families, they propose that these different parental styles may impact differently on the developing brain. Working class parenting styles are suggested to be more detrimental, and this is proposed to add another layer – and further confirmation – of Lareau's original insights that these differing parental styles of engagement in children's education prepared children differently for adulthood, in some cases reinforcing inequalities. Middle class parents' 'concerted cultivation' resulted in children focusing on skills and education development, thus better equipping them for school and for higher education. In contrast, working class parents were seen to take a more permissive approach ('natural growth'), trusting their children to develop in their own ways. McEwen and McEwen appear to imply that the working class approach to parenting is also associated with toxic stress, which seems quite a leap to make. They suggest that 'research ... needs to tease out the social sources of variability in parenting in early childhood among low-income households and within low-income neighbourhoods' (p 463). This ignores the numerous studies which have examined parenting in diverse settings, and social sources of such variability are well understood within childhood and youth studies, and education (Cooper, 2020; Holloway and Pimlott-Wilson, 2014). These studies highlight the vital role of material inequality itself in shaping parenting styles (and educational outcomes). Other studies have examined the role of trauma and violence in shaping parenting styles (Cluver et al, 2020) – an important qualifier, since McEwen and McEwen's paper seems to slip between suggesting that certain forms of traumatic childhood experience cause 'toxic stress' and implying that all forms of working class parenting may cause such problems.

There are significant dangers in interdisciplinary collaborations – with the potential that insights from each discipline may be lost at unfortunate points. McEwen and McEwen's paper epitomizes such slippages, where assumptions about 'good parenting' are made which are inherently (middle) classed, but not recognized as such; and where 'toxicity' is attached to parenting style, rather than to class cultures and the oppressive structural contexts in which many families struggle. But fundamentally, why do we require neurobiological evidence of harm caused by apparently 'toxic' stress? (see also Rose, 2018). This brings us face-to-face with a range of limits to the stress paradigm, which we expand on in the next section.

Limits of the stress paradigm

To many scholars, the stress paradigm constitutes a useful generic frame to research mental health. However, it has limitations.

In a 2017 overview of the field, Thoits sets out three key limitations. First, she notes that the paradigm does not explain individual cases of psychological disorder, being better suited for group-based predictions. Second, existing work on stress does not explain variation in *responses* to stressful situations, for instance, why studies find higher rates of depressive symptoms among women, and higher use of alcohol and drugs among men, and so forth. Finally, the stress paradigm does not explain all disorders well. Echoing debates led by Horwitz (2007), Thoits suggests that when it comes to psychosis in particular, other explanatory factors, particularly relating to genes, neurochemistry or childhood socialization, may play more important roles. All this resonates with long-standing debates within the sociology of mental health as to what the appropriate focus of our subdiscipline should be when it comes to aetiology or causation. This is a fascinating example of the way in which the sociology of mental health sometimes splits off particular areas of human life (such as psychosis) and apportions them as 'non-social' and therefore of less interest for sociological explanation and analysis.[3]

Surprisingly, beyond these 'secondary' limitations, the assumptions underlying the stress paradigm have remained approximately the same since Selye. Why would stress be *the* 'core emotion' or process explaining distress and mental disorder – and why not others? What allows us to formalize social life to such extent, separating in all contexts some 'stressors', 'buffers' and (objective or perceived) 'stress'? What is the social and psychological evidence for such a reduction? These narratives are rarely questioned, and despite the scientific tone often adopted by proponents of the stress paradigm, this paradigm is based on fragile, taken-for-granted assumptions that can, and must, be troubled. We identify five problematic stances within studies aligned with the stress paradigm: the universality of stress; the measurability of stress; the abstraction of context; moral conservatism and the lack of novel findings.

Universality of stress

One of the strengths of the stress paradigm is that by centring its theory of mental disorders on a common, universal, concept – stress – it enables the gathering of an extraordinary amount of data, whose analyses can accumulate and strengthen the model. Stress has been used to account for the difficulties experienced by Russian people transitioning to new ways of life following the dissolution of the USSR (Union of Soviet Socialist Republics, Pietila and Rytkonen, 2008), and for forms of distress specifically found among Peruvian agriculturalists, *chucaque* (Brooks, 2014), or Mexican people, *nervios* and *susto* (Weller et al, 2008). Elsewhere, poverty is framed as a chronic stressor enabling policies to be revised in terms of stress reduction (Hjelm et al, 2017), while the adversity of cultural adaptation in migrants can be re-branded as 'acculturative stress' (Chartonas and Bose, 2015). Supposedly based on common biological features, *stress* comes to constitute an all-purpose word that captures core emotional processes, depicting the malaise of every citizen of the world. In fact, using the stress paradigm requires reframing social life – no matter its context – as made of potentially 'stressful social arrangements' (Horwitz, 2007) depending on 'environmental adversity' (Dohrenwend, 2000), with 'stressors' on one side, 'stress-buffering mechanisms' or 'protective factors' on the other.

But is stress a universal prism to understand the motor of distress? Are all the experiences mentioned above *of the same kind*? If yes, what can prove this? (We have not found any evidence in the literature.) As per Jackson's (2013) study, stress is situated in a history. The very word 'stress' has one. A quick search on *Google Ngram*[4] shows that the use of this word rose throughout the twentieth century in English-speaking literature to peak in the 1980s, while it circulated from English to other languages, such as French and Italian, in the second half of the same century. As Schwartz (2011) notes about French bus drivers, the psychological lexicon, its international and inter-class diffusion (from the upper to the working class) can be ethnographically monitored, traced back to the 1980s diffusion of the 'psychological mass culture' in France, which entails growing inclinations – or even dispositions – to interpret daily tensions in terms of stress.

These observations point to the importance of understanding the *inextricable* relation between stress as a transcendent dimension of human life, and 'stress' as a cultural idiom (all the more, an Anglicism) circulating in globalized societies.

Measurability of stress

In much of the research that develops the stress process model, 'objective' measures of stress primarily 'rely on the assumption that standardized items mean the same things to members of different groups' (McLeod, 2012, p 177). However, McLeod argues, it is well understood that the way in which people make sense of and interpret their 'objective' life experiences is shaped by their social position and the 'ideologies' they may have as resources through which to interpret their experiences (p 179). Similarly, Williams (2018, p 467) notes that '[h]istorically, the assessment of stressful life experiences was heavily driven by the stressors experienced by middle class white males'; which means that the stress of 'other' groups – women, sexual, racial, ethnic and religious minority groups – has been measured a posteriori, without consideration of their specific experiences; by extension identified relationships between exposure to 'stressors' and mental health outcomes may poorly represent diverse social groups (Meyer, 2003; Varcoe et al, 2019). To be clear, this problem is not overcome by studies highlighting the subjectivity and inequality of stress, since the issue is not only to understand *how* various groups make sense of different levels of stress, but *whether and to what extent* this notion applies to them (Valdez et al, 2013; Wadman et al, 2018), especially when they use different words such as *nervios*.

Another foundational assumption of the stress paradigm is that the events, processes and emotions at stake in the genesis of mental disorders are measurable. As McLeod (2012) notes, there are two ways of measuring this, common to qualitative and quantitative methods:

- Directly – asking participants how stressed they are.
- Indirectly – inferring from certain experiences how stressed participants are; for instance, how divorce affects the likeliness to be diagnosed with depression.

The indirect technique includes a significant risk of over-interpretation: how do we know that if a correlation exists between divorce and depression, it is because divorces are stressful? More direct approaches inherently risk an imposition bias, since inquiring about stress incites participants to use this frame – especially questionnaires that do not include opportunity to elaborate on this notion or propose one's own words instead. Even cortisol measurements do not solve the problem; they indicate a certain level of tension 'in the body', but their association with stress remains subject to much debate in medical research (Roberts and McWade, 2021) – sociological studies have long showed that the same substance does not mechanically lead to the same effects and meanings (Becker, 1963).

Another methodological issue appears if we turn to the 'outcomes' of stress, distress and/or mental disorders. Horwitz (2007) and Schwartz (2007) note that both outcomes are often merged. Whereas some studies that focus on the relationship between stressful experiences and development of diagnosable 'mental disorders' clearly characterize what they mean by mental illness

(Webb et al, 2017), a significant proportion of stress research is concerned with more diffuse experiences of distress. Some argue that experiences of 'distress' should be regarded as 'normal' and not equated with the experience of 'disorder' which should be deemed 'abnormal' (Horwitz, 2007; Wheaton, 2007). Various measures were also designed to identify 'distress' as a result of 'stressors' (Aneshensel, 2015; Scott et al, 2018). But more deeply, all these works share the assumption that a continuum of measurable, progressive states transcend human life: stress → distress → mental disorder. The problem being, nothing proves that this process exists in all humans rather than as a by-product of methodological procedures.

Further, measures vary widely. Often presented as reflecting the state of research or some logical knowledge, they can often be tied to assumptions made by researchers about what constitutes distress, and indeed mental disorder. Some use survey instruments such as the Patient Health Questionnaire-9 and take high scores for specific disorders such as depression, anxiety or post-traumatic stress disorder (PTSD) as evidence of distress (Mersky et al, 2018). Other studies use self-reported symptoms of what may be understood by lay people as 'stress' but are operationalized so as to be measurable outcomes of stress – feeling overwhelmed, experiencing tremors or shaking (Fothergill et al, 2016). In our view – echoing Wheaton (2007), Mirowsky (2007) and others – debates about whether these studies are comparable or measuring 'the same thing' rather miss the point. We know that what is labelled as a 'disorder', 'normal' or 'abnormal' 'distress' is highly contingent and culturally variable.

Thus it becomes urgent to reorient the stress paradigm towards less imperialist forms of understanding that, no matter which methodology is employed, properly reflects the diversity of distressing emotions and disorders found in societies and individuals.

Abstraction of context

A third feature of much research aligned to the stress paradigm is the tendency to abstract context – often necessary in order to operationalize measurements of 'stressors'. In a contribution to the *Handbook for the Study of Mental Health*, Thoits framed the entire subdiscipline of the sociology of mental health around 'factors external to the individual ... causing a breakdown in the face of overwhelming environmental *stress*' (Thoits, 2017, emphasis added). The field would be uniquely concerned with 'the stressful consequences of social organization rather than the stressful antecedents of psychological disorder' (Aneshensel, 1992, p 15). However, much sociological work on stress does a fairly poor job of conceptualizing and engaging with social worlds, which Thoits (1995, p 52) also acknowledges: 'Despite attributions of the origins of stress to large-scale social structures or processes few investigators have attempted to examine the links between macrolevel factors and microlevel experiences.' Instead *social* factors are translated into concerns with ultimately *individual* responses to and resources against disadvantage, such as coping resources or how people can access services depending on their economic and geographical situations. Schwartz (2002) observes this trend in some sociologists' reliance on psychological constructs such as mastery or self-esteem; a focus on quantifying negative events, positive relationships; or an individualistic focus on how individuals might 'cope' with adversity.

The way that different groups of people respond to 'stressors' may in itself be socially variable, and this must be an ongoing area of study for sociologists interested in the relationship between society, stress and disorder: an approach that allows for engagement with interpretive and expressive processes – attached to 'stress' but not only – which are entangled with meaning as well as social and political structures (McLeod, 2012; Thomas et al, 2020).

Also, let us note the focus on 'coping' and the role that sociology might have in identifying why some groups apparently navigate stressors more 'successfully' (with fewer negative mental health 'outcomes'), and in proposing 'interventions' to support those who experience poorer outcomes. Many studies, for instance, explore the role of 'coping resources' in mediating identified relationships between stressors and negative outcomes. However, such coping resources are often framed as something that people have or do not have, that they require 'training' or 'education' to help them acquire – drawing on deficit models. As a consequence, even if the stress paradigm theoretically puts emphasis on social or structural variables, its conclusions are often individual in practice. Studies might propose 'intensive pre-schooling' for children who have spent their early years in poverty, for instance (McEwen and McEwen, 2017, p 458). Such approaches side-step the issue of poverty itself, and focus – perhaps pragmatically, given the political climate in the US and UK – on interventions aiming to 'break the cycle' of poverty on an individual or family level (see Macdonald et al, 2013 for a critique of such approaches).

Moral conservatism

The fourth feature we propose as a limitation of the stress paradigm is a tendency towards moral conservatism. In the stress model, what is stressful is negative while what is not stressful is positive. Hans Selye himself was surprised by the anti-stress stance his work has inspired. In response he recalled in a later publication that stress remains the *'spice of life'*!

The assumption that stress, or too much stress, is inherently negative has moral and political connotations, mainly because social and personal changes are stressful. For instance, many studies suggest that changes in the realms of work or family are detrimental to mental health. Barrett and Turner (2005) show higher levels of depression in 'stepfamilies, single parent families, and single parent families with other relatives present, compared with mother-father families' (p 156). Without asserting any moral standpoint about family forms, these conclusions still re-enact the healthiness of traditional (or unchanging/stable) lifestyles, since they avoid two important issues. First, it is a 'normal' dimension of social change to feel more stressed in an atypical or transitional situation: are not experiments, by definition, more stressful than what is already known? Living in an 'alternative' household might be stressful, and even provoke mental distress, but approaches in terms of stress forget the broader 'positive' aspects change might bring – for which stress might be worth experiencing. Second, at a societal level, the status quo is often less stressful than change. Keeping the same lifestyle, political and economic system might well be more relaxing, for some at least. Research has suggested that revolutionaries in France (Murat, 2014) and the US (see Metzl, 2010 on civil rights activists) were over-represented in psychiatric wards. Struggling for change – contributing to civil rights activism, coming out, declaring one's sexual abuse, challenging traditions – are stressful endeavours. It might additionally attract the scrutiny of powerful others, who may seek to pathologize such struggles.

A related point returns us to the recommendations of much research in the stress paradigm, which proposes that it may be more straightforward to give people 'coping skills' than it is to change the circumstances of their lives. While not wishing to dismiss a desire to help and to reduce negative outcomes among groups who face more challenges, there are dangers in going too far down this path alone. Such paths can result in an ultimately individualistic foc us of stress, coping and resources among individuals (Varcoe et al, 2019), resulting in a 'toothless' sociology (Tyler, 2020, p 100) which – inadvertently or not – results in blaming the victims, and raises significant questions about 'whose side we are on' (Becker, 1967). A simple illustration of this comes from the policies implemented regarding stress among dominated groups, such as women and indigenous people, in former or current colonizing countries. There is a significant – inseparably *political and psychological* – gap between teaching coping resources to individuals (offering meditation lessons and free therapy), resistance behaviours (self-defence lessons and legal training) or addressing the roots of the problem (such as gender stereotypes and land rights) (see Ansloos and Peltier, 2021, and X and polanco, 2021 for analysis of these issues in relation to suicide).

All in all, some conservative, or at least individualistic, moral assumptions can be identified, and thus, putting the concept of stress at the core of a theory or programme of research is far from neutral, 'scientific' or based on biology. As with any paradigm, the stress paradigm carries a social and political philosophy, and remaining ignorant of this is detrimental to its validity.

Lack of novel findings

Our final concern with the stress paradigm is — perhaps surprisingly — a lack of novel findings. What do we know better after three decades of increasingly expansive research drawing on this stress? Has this research perspective helped us discover things that we did not know before? Relative to the considerable amount of works and publications it has generated, the stress paradigm has been relatively unproductive in generating novel outcomes. To put it bluntly: when people are stressed, they are more likely to feel distressed and to experience mental health issues; poorer people and people from stigmatized minority groups are exposed to more stress. Some exceptions exist, as stressful professions (doctors and lawyers) have high levels of reported stress; and some resources help people deal with stress, such as having a family, financial means, social support networks and stability. Some nuances can be found as well — that in certain contexts, certain variables have slightly different weights in palliating stress. Of course, the purpose of this paradigm was to turn these common sense ideas into academic research designs where statistical correlations, and discourses (for qualitative methods), enhance understanding of how the social dimensions of stress arise and intersect with mental health. Still, many reasonings in the literature remain tautological in the sense that they examine the stressful nature of things that are already known to be stressful.

For instance, higher status professions such as lawyers and doctors face considerable responsibility and work long hours; divorces are considered to be a failure in societies valuing marriage; financial instability is difficult as money facilitates access to most items enabling survival and comfort; chronic illness requires constant medical monitoring and health uncertainty. These are obvious and expected conclusions; however, key findings of the stress paradigm proponents include that some high-status people are stressed, divorce provokes stress, financial instability and chronic illness are stressors. In other words, the stress model (as any theory) runs the risk of creating a self-sufficient world that generates its own questions and for which common sense answers appear path-breaking because they add to the model.

In the following two sections we introduce two directions for research and theorization which draws on — but moves beyond — the stress paradigm. The first of these concerns stressful dominations: how relations of oppression, domination and power shape stressful experiences and responses to such experiences. The second considers how we can draw on the sociology of emotions to diversify and add nuance to our understanding of how such experiences play out in more complex ways than captured by 'stress'.

Stressful dominations

How do inequalities relating to intersecting social identities and positions shape experiences and responses to stress? In this section we consider how approaches that take social inequalities and diversity seriously further expand the more linear processes implied in the orthodox formulations of the stress model. The role of intersectionality (Crenshaw, 1991; Bowleg, 2008; Collins and Bilge, 2016) is key here, as the social world is not a blank page on which quantities of stress carry equal weight and generate the same meanings in all locations.

Recent scholarship has sought to engage with the stratified and intersectional nature of stress, and better understand how social inequalities turn into health inequalities. For instance, attempts have been made to examine racism and oppression of sexual and racial minorities as a source of stress (Williams, 2018), such as the 'minority stress' argument, according to which racial, social and ethnic minorities suffer from a particular type of stress associated with discrimination (Meyer, 2003; Schmitz et al, 2019). As per Chapter 1, the leading conclusion is: in most cases,[5] the lower people are in a social hierarchy, the more exposed to stress they are and the less resources to buffer it they possess (Longest and Thoits, 2012; Turner, 2013).

In the sociology of mental health, these approaches emerged around social psychological reflections regarding the unequal opportunities to 'let off steam'. Horwitz, for instance, drawing on early work by Mirowsky (1985) suggests that one explanation for the greater levels of stress among people inhabiting positions of less power relates to emotional expression.

> In general, mental health should vary directly with domination and inversely with subordination in systems of social relationships. Dominants can express feelings toward subordinates more freely and so can vent frustrations and aggressions openly in a downward direction. Subordinates, however, are much more limited in their capacity to vent emotions upward and so would be more likely to express them through signs of depression, anxiety, or psychophysiological symptoms that do not directly confront the dominant party. (Horwitz, 2002, p 173)

The repression of emotions in this theoretical position is causally associated with the development of '(di)stress': 'dependents must often internalize hostile emotions and consequently develop physiological or neurotic symptoms' (Horwitz, 2002, p 173). Horwitz' support for this assertion draws on two studies of power, gender and distress, each of which focuses on women's differing responses to strain in heterosexual marriage (Horwitz, 1982; Levy, 1976).

In the next sections we further expand on the idea of stress as inherently generated within the web of social dominations that structures societies, partly through emotional repression and expression. This way of understanding stress is exemplified in two broad approaches: (a) a focus on *differentiated socialization*, where different social groups – particularly along lines of gender – are socialized in ways which may generate more stress and inhibit the expression of distress in ways which further enhance likelihood of mental illness; and (b) *minority stress* perspectives, which underline a special type of stress generated by being a member of a social group that is routinely marginalized or discredited.

Socialization to stress

In this reasoning, not only do social inequalities produce different levels of stress, but also shape the meanings of stress in relation to different social positions, shaping how stress – or other emotions – are expressed. Stress is thus entangled in the socialization process, and the social roles that different groups inhabit.

Gender has attracted particular attention in this regard. Developing gender role theory (Gove and Tudor, 1973), Simon (2020, 2002) interprets differences in men and women's accounts of mental health in the US in light of gender identity: crucially, women's greater levels of distress could be understood in part through their greater perceived tensions between work and family/household responsibilities. These tensions were less present, or absent, for men, who by virtue of their gender are far less likely to be held responsible for either care of children or a household. Despite significant advances in women's rights and position in society, childcare and household management continue to be highly gendered practices, with associated implications for the meanings that upset or unhappiness in either domain may cause for men and women (Simon, 2020; Sullivan et al, 2018).

A frequent suggestion across the sociology of mental health (and beyond) is that men and women differ in how they express stress.

> Males tend to predominate among disorders involving outward-turning behaviors, including acting against others, while females tend to predominate in disorders characterized by inward-turning behaviors involving self-blame and internal upset. (Turner et al, 2007, p 79)

These gendered understandings of stress may reflect gendered ways of experiencing emotions more generally (Lupton, 1998). However, as with much in the simplistic world of binary gender, on closer inspection this dualistic model becomes less clear. For instance, while women (or subordinates) are associated more often with repression, anxiety and depression, in some cultural imaginaries it is *men* who are associated with emotional repression ('boys don't cry' and the 'stiff upper lip' in the UK). In such cases men are expected to maintain a 'rational', 'objective' emotionality, associated with masculinity (not femininity); whereas emotional 'outbursts' (albeit not angry or violent) are associated with *femininity* (not masculinity) (de Boise and Hearn, 2017; Lupton, 1998).

Emotions infuse theories of how stressors are understood to impact on individuals, but also via their responses to stressors. In terms of gender, men's responses to stressors via violence/aggression ('outward-turning behaviours') are made possible because of their 'dominant' position, which makes such expressions socially acceptable – and in some instances encouraged (de Boise and Hearn, 2017). Similarly, Longest and Thoits (2012) suggest that adherence to 'traditional female gender roles' among many women and some men may explain particular configurations of stress (a tendency to internalize); this rests in part on the idea that traditional female gender roles inhibit externalization of distress, whereas some 'nontraditional women' and more 'traditional men' will externalize distress.

This raises questions, though, about whether men (or indeed 'nontraditional women') responding to stressors via aggression should be understood as 'stressed' in the same way that women responding to stressors via internalizing disorders should be understood as 'stressed'. They may sometimes experience similar stressors, but this research suggests strongly that the 'same' stressors are not experienced in the same way, and that the different modes of emotionality, aligned with gender in these cases, provoke different trajectories or outcomes. Bluntly, the argument is that women's 'internalization' of stress contributes to greater diagnoses of depression and anxiety. They 'repress' stress and it 'produces' disorder (Busfield, 1996).

The case of suicide and self-harm opens an interesting angle on this issue. It is unclear – and there is some inconsistency – as to whether self-harm and/or suicide represent 'internalizing' or 'externalizing' of (di)stress. Certainly, both self-harm and suicide are understood and described as responses to 'stressors'. Gendered assumptions appear to shape how these practices are interpreted. For instance, while suicide is sometimes referred to as an 'internalizing' expression of self-blame or shame (see Stack, 2000, on race and suicide), when discussing men and women's differing rates of suicide and self-harm it is self-harm that becomes a sign of 'internalizing' distress, while suicide becomes an 'externalizing' expression (see Chandler, 2019, and discussion below). In a recent study, Chandler and Simopoulou (2021), drawing on Jaworski (2014), raised serious questions about how both self-harm and suicide are understood as gendered, especially questioning the common interpretation of self-harm as a 'feminine', 'internalizing' act. Other qualitative studies have demonstrated the complexity of suicide (and self-harm) and indicate that we should be cautious when resorting to simplistic binarisms when considering social life (Whynacht, 2018; Steggals et al, 2020).

In sum, any expression of mental distress and disorder is *already* gendered (Busfield, 1996); therefore, the association between stress and gender, as the example of suicide/self-harm shows, implies not only considering traditional gender expectations and how they relate to gendered types of emotions, but also questioning how *interpretations* of these emotions, and the associated behaviours and disorders, are gendered.

This drives us back to the problem of measurement. A major challenge within stress research is that groups found to have higher levels of stress/distress may instead reflect that stress/distress is being more readily identified among those groups (whether by researchers, or by study participants themselves). For instance, Longest and Thoits' (2012) analysis, above, suggests that 'nontraditional men' may constitute the majority of 'distressed men' in their study, suggesting perhaps something about a feminine/female role that invites distress or – conversely – that distress is itself read as feminine and female (Busfield, 1996). Meyer, for example, has hypothesized that the higher rates of distress reported among gay, bisexual and lesbian groups may relate to their having a lower threshold for recognizing and articulating symptoms (Schwartz and Meyer, 2010).

The relationship between power, social structure and emotion is further unsettled when considering racial or ethnic minorities. As discussed previously, the relationship between race, ethnicity and mental disorder is complex, and subject to challenges with measurement and meaning (Williams, 2018). Enrolling race and ethnicity in understanding variations in stress, along with the meanings of different forms of emotionality (repression, expression, anger, anxiety) challenges binary ways of thinking about male/female emotionality and disorder. Returning to suicide, Chandler (2019) noted that explanations for the lower rates of suicide found among African American men, compared to white men in the US, drew on related ideas of domination, internalization and externalization (Stack, 2000). In this case, white men are framed as the social group that 'internalizes' distress, because they are the dominant group so cannot blame others for their 'failings'. African American men, in contrast may 'blame others' and externalize their distress in violence against others. This interpretation of the meaning of suicide problematically ignores rates of non-fatal self-harm, and it subverts usual notions of (all) men as tending to 'externalize' their distress in order to account for one of the 'paradoxes' of mental health – that in this case the 'subordinate' group (African American men) are not killing themselves at expected levels (unlike Native American men, who die by suicide at rates higher than any other).

Thus, depending on their social position – gender, class, race and so on – people are socialized differently to emotions, exposed to various explanatory discourses about their distress, and to different expressions of stress that are socially gendered, racialized, classed, and so forth. If today these inequalities are well understood, how socializations to stress occur in different groups and in *historically constituted forms* remain relatively uncharted territory. A good example is provided by the (stressful) dominations that Native Americans, Asians, Arabs, Latinos and African Americans suffer from in the US, whose construction and continued enactment (Wolfe, 2016) differ at least for the historical reasons (colonization, slavery, long-term or recent economic migrations, geopolitical events) that delineate each group's perceived and actual social situation – with not solely *unequal* but *differing* effects on lifecourse, meaning and mental health 'outcomes' like suicide. This points again to the importance of meaning in understanding how stress may emerge from particular social configurations. The meaning of what it is to be a member of a minoritized ethnic group (and of a certain gender) and its emotional consequences are embedded in each context; this is another aspect of 'socialization to stress'.

Minority stress

Building on the above, Meyer's (2003) concept of 'minority stress' offers an approach which *does* centre meaning. Meyer is concerned with the way in which social interactions between members of groups who are classed as 'minorities' – minority ethnic groups or those who identify as LGBTQ+ – and others can generate stress that accumulates for members of minority groups. This model incorporates less easily 'objectively identified' causes of stress, such as a more diffuse experience of feeling 'out of place', of having one's identity regularly misrecognized or castigated in social interactions (there are parallels here with Ahmed's *Queer Phenomenology*, 2006). Minority stress provides a potentially productive way of identifying and engaging with experiences of prejudice and discrimination as generators of stress, as well as the more diffuse experience of unease and discomfort that may emerge from inhabiting a social context where one's identity is the subject of negative, invalidating responses.

The concept of minority stress offers some ways forward for considering the intersecting nature of social identities and positions, with sociocultural meanings remaining central. Meyer (2003) provides a number of examples to illustrate this. Noting that, for instance, experiences of discrimination on the basis of sexual identity have been found to vary, he cites a study by Krieger and Sidney (1997, in Meyer, 2003) which found that one third of African American gay adults reported incidents of discrimination, compared to one half of white adults. Meyer contrasts this, though, with another study by Siegal and Epstein (1996, in Meyer, 2003) which found that experiences of discrimination among HIV+ men in New York were more frequently described by African American and Puerto Rican men than by white men. These few examples indicate that stress is unequally produced in societies and that minorities face specific issues in this regard.[6]

Further, discrimination may also be *experienced* differently: the meanings and implications of minor and major acts of discrimination may be more keenly felt by some, even within the same groups. As Meyer points out, one of the challenges of minority stress theories is to effectively explain the finding that in some cases minority ethnic groups have lower rates of mental disorder (or suicide, as we saw above). As Williams (2018) notes, challenges with measuring and identifying 'disorder' among different racial, ethnic and cultural groups underlie this mystery.[7] Meyer suggests that a crucial difference between LGBT groups and, for instance, black/African American groups is that the latter are more likely to be 'born into' a community, within which they may grow up and develop positive meanings associated with membership of such community. In contrast, in most cases LGBT people acquire their identity later in life, and may face additional stresses related to 'coming out' or negative responses from the families or communities they grew up with. To build on the discussion above, though, this argument does not hold well when applied to indigenous groups in settler-colonial countries where – even within 'communities' – rates of mental disorder and suicide are high (Wexler, 2006; Gone, 2013).

This resonates with wider findings in the sociology of stress, according to which 'identity-salient' stressors have more impact (Thoits, 2013). Thus, social identity – gender, race/ethnicity, sexuality – may expose individuals to different types of stress, but may also affect how they respond to the same stressors. Central here is the meaning – mediated by social identity – of different stressors. For instance, Simon (2020) suggests that women are more negatively impacted than men by the stress of caring for a disabled or chronically ill child, as their social position generally enrols them in more of the day-to-day care, but further, Simon argues that their social identity as mothers (rather than fathers) leads them to be far more affected by the health status of their children. Similarly, women in dual-earner couples report greater levels of stress and distress because of the very different cultural meanings which women navigate in such situations in comparison to men: women blame themselves for not spending enough time with children, and experience greater strain between the roles of worker and mother. Again, despite advances in women's rights and labour market participation, cultural meanings relating to women and motherhood, and men and fatherhood, continue to construct these roles differently, with different implications for stress and mental disorder (Simon, 2020).

Stigma is, of course, deeply connected to the concept of minority stress – the negative attributes that are associated with particular social identities, especially in relation to sexuality, stand at the core of this social process through which minorities experience more stress, or a different kind of stress. Recent work on the sociology of stigma has further developed an analysis of stigma in relation to poverty and class (Scambler, 2018; Shildrick, 2018; Thomas et al, 2020; Tyler, 2020) that offers a vital way of elaborating the 'stress process' model by incorporating meaning. The stress process model already implicates the stresses and strains of poverty, issues such as struggling to pay bills, sourcing adequate food, living in disordered neighbourhoods with high rates of crime, and living in poor housing. Attending to the additional stresses of inhabiting a stigmatized identity in relation to class position, economic status or the place that people live, in contexts where stigma can be politically used to blame certain categories of the population or institutionalized through policies, provides an additional manner of approaching how social configurations shape incidence of mental disorder beyond the generic, individualizing model of stress charactering the stress paradigm (we return to stigma in Chapter 3).

These insights underline that stress is not a process that can be straightforwardly 'measured in' various fractions of the population, unquestionably compared among these fractions as different amounts of the same thing. Rather, its reality is conditioned by meanings, socializations and inequalities that change its very nature and relationship to mental disorder. This is why some minority groups might experience specific forms of stress given their singular situation in societies shaped by intersecting forms of oppression. Whether addressing stress, emotions or any idiom of distress, these nuances and variations raise awareness of the differential impact of relationships to power and domination, and need to be accounted for in any sociological understanding of the social genesis of mental disorders.

From the meaning of stress to the sociology of emotions

Can all the emotional processes involved in the emergence of mental disorders be reasonably summarized as underlain by a form of 'stress'? In view of the multiplicity, complexity and variability of social situations reported by sociologists, historians and anthropologists of mental health and emotions, the definitive answer is no.

A long tradition in social sciences and philosophy addresses the entanglement between capitalism, relations of domination and emotional experiences at the core of mental disorders. For example, merging the Freudian legacy and critical theory, the Frankfurt School notably explored this path. Marcuse's (1974) notion of repressive surplus typically 'sociologizes' Freudian psychoanalysis to contest the view that humans would repress their emotions for the common good, out of natural necessity; instead, they control themselves for the perpetuation of economic production, capital accumulation and traditional social orders. Elias (2000) made the case that emotions and their social/intimate management result from long-term power dynamics. The increasing size of interdependence networks, the shifting modes of exercise of power and geopolitical dynamics more broadly socialized people to self-regulation. More recent elaborations include cultural understandings of emotion, such as Lupton's (1998) view on emotional repression in relation to Freudian concepts of neuroticism or anxiety, thought to result from excessive repression of subconscious (often sexual) 'impulses'. Lupton identified, among lay people in twentieth century Australia, common articulations of emotional 'health' which similarly rested on ideas about unruly emotions, and the need to both 'release' these but also 'control' them.

This is an ongoing challenge for the sociology of mental health, the stress paradigm or any other perspectives destined to replace it: contextualizing the emotional processes underpinning the emergence of mental distress in such a way that the considerable variation of emotions, produced and interpreted in given socio-political contexts, is accounted for. Works like that of Castel (2012) sketch how this can be realized from a historical perspective, showing that the succession of trends in Western psychology – psychoanalysis, then behavioural psychology and neuropsychology – mirror broader contexts where the guilt of repressed desires (which made the heyday of psychoanalysis) were overrun by a collective, aspirational notion of the autonomous self (which enabled behavioural psychology to flourish, and later approaches centred on the brain). This modified the very form of obsessions and anxieties in the West. In anthropology, Jenkins (2015) offered an in-depth account of how to read various mental illnesses through contextualized emotions and culture, reading the experience of antipsychotic drugs among psychotic patients in 2000s California to trauma among Salvadorian refugees in 1980s Boston.

We should merge the stress paradigm with the sociology, anthropology and history of emotions. This idea is not new. Receiving the Leonard Pearlin Award,[8] Schieman (2019) supported greater integration between sociologies of stress, mental health and emotion. This stance entails more explicit and critical engagement with how emotions are enrolled in imaginaries about stress and mental disorder, as well as the crucial role of social structures and cultures in shaping emotional experience and expression (Lupton, 1998). These connections should also be empirically articulated, using an array of methods which can reflect the contingent, culturally variable and socially shaped nature of emotions. The sociology of emotions does not assume a common element in the experience of all mental disorders (stress) but instead takes the particularities of emotional experiences as a starting point, which opens ways of studying, for instance, ADHD through anger (Singh, 2011), anorexia through 'abjection' (Warin, 2010) or historically understanding depression as the medicalization of sadness (Horwitz, 2011). Such approaches also open opportunities to further tie these emotional experiences with their sociohistorical contexts, as Orr (2006) does with panic disorders in the US, analysing the cultural construction of 'panic' as an affect embedded in both 'psychopower' and US politics surrounding outside threats.

In the following paragraphs, we sketch some lines of inquiry based on the examination of two emotional idioms often encountered in accounts of mental illness: anger and paranoia.

Anger!

'Assaultive or Belligerent?' This question tops a 1970s promotional poster for Haldol, an antipsychotic drug, in the US. Below the title, the drawing of a black man, furiously raising his left fist, is paired with the apparent, pharmaceutical, resolution: 'Cooperation often begins with Haldol'. Metzl (2010, p xiv) uses this poster to illustrate a phenomenon that long preoccupied psychiatrists: why so many black men are diagnosed with and treated for psychotic disorders. Metzl argues that understanding this cannot be separated from broader social concerns – racism, and resistance to racism. As in the deeply problematic Haldol advert, what might otherwise be understood as rationally indignant responses to oppression and inequity are interpreted by (white) psychiatrists as evidencing aggression, disrespect and individuals or populations being out of (white) control. This 'problem', Metzl notes, particularly soared after the Second World War at a time when a proportion of these black men regularly took to the streets, a phenomenon otherwise known as the civil rights movement. This brings us to the question: under which social conditions is anger deemed pathological?

Some of the most serious mental disorders involve outbursts of *anger*. In the DSM-5 (American Psychiatric Association, 2013) more than 30 items include, in their symptomatology, forms of aggressivity or irritability. A few disorders even centre these emotions, such as Intermittent Explosive Disorder and Oppositional Defiant Disorder. These disorders – and the problematization of anger – might be understood in light of Elias' (2000) 'civilising process' where, over centuries, Westerners are allegedly expected to be calmer, with greater control over their emotions. Anger threatens the functioning of schools, workplaces, families, local communities. Therefore, anger as a potential symptom cannot be read individually: it expresses a relation to various social orders.

Moreover, unpacking anger in context can offer further ways of understanding the social experience of mental health issues. In their research of a facility for adolescents in New Mexico, Jenkins and Csordas (2020, pp 130–161) dedicate a chapter to anger. This emotion, they explain, was referenced by more than half of their participants as central to their lived experience of mental illness. Jenkins and Csordas detail how two adolescents, one girl and one boy, communicated their experience of mental illness *through* how they feel anger in their social life – what upsets them in their family, at school and, then, in the hospital. Very importantly, anger is also a moral emotion. An hospital staff member comments: 'there is a lot to be angry about in today's world, … so maybe it is a healthy sign' (Jenkins and Csordas, 2020, p 152). In raising such ambivalence, Jenkins and Csordas frame anger as a component of some experiences of mental illness, both as a disruptive emotion in everyday life and an understandable, if not healthy, form of awareness.

In addition, the experience of anger (in relation to mental health) varies depending on the social divides in which people and groups are located. Alang's (2016) ethnographic research in a poor, predominantly African American community in the Midwest of the US, found anger was a common way in which depression was expressed. Alang's study offers an important intervention whereby experiences of mental illness can be understood as situated within a particular social context – shaped by racial and socioeconomic disadvantage, by local meanings and attitudes towards health and ill-health – each of which can be seen to inter-relate. Using a quantitative measurement of stress would miss that what matters here is the historically and socially constructed meaning of 'anger' and its discrepant (and differently stressful) appropriation in social stratification.

Elsewhere, drawing on survey research in Florida, measuring 'violent adversities', 'chronic strains', 'discrimination stress' and 'anger proneness', Turner et al (2007) found that reported experiences of anger vary by gender as well as by socioeconomic status: among young women, those who had fewer economic resources were more likely to report 'short tempered anger'. They conclude that these findings

> support the crucial hypothesis that anger proneness is at least partially conditioned by social experience and context. If this is accepted, it follows that such proneness is potentially preventable or modifiable through interventions aimed at reducing stress exposure and enhancing the availability of social and personal resources over the early life course. (Turner et al, 2007, p 79)

These conclusions echo those proposed by McEwen and McEwen (2017) in focusing on the potential for 'interventions' to disrupt the relationship between social experiences (violence) and context (poverty), and later anger and mental disorder;[9] rather than addressing *why* particular adversities may be found among certain social groups and positions. In the face of such intractable stressors (or causes of anger), this focus on intervention ultimately individualizes emotions and attempt to inculcate individual 'buffers', rather than looking at collective and political transformations which would reduce oppression, marginalization and powerlessness in the first place.

Further questions arise when questioning whether anger is inherently 'bad' — or reflecting on the 'function' of anger. In his ethnography of crack dealers in 1990s Harlem, Bourgois (1995) portrays how one of his participants regularly manifested outbursts of rage and that this contributed to him presenting a self that was unpredictable and 'crazy'. Far from being discrediting (nobody dared suggest therapy) this young man used this representation to scare his clients and competitors: a matter of survival in the violent world of crack dealers. This example is instructive. It reveals that considering stress and anger as potentially pathological *without contextualizing such processes* equates to naturalizing a Western middle class representation of the world, where society is pacified enough — supposedly — for stress and anger to occur as personal problems.

Anger can be understood as the feeling of injustice. Conducting interviews with West Papuan refugees in Australia, Rees and Silove (2011) inquire into Sakit Hati, a 'culture-bound syndrome' close to amok, showing how this disorder expresses resentment, ultimately pointing to human rights violations. Anger here manifests a relation to the political situation of Papua New Guinea — and asylum policies in Australia — *as much as* it formulates individual feelings. If emotions cannot be detached from their context, then the study of their pathologization should also address the conditions of their emergence.

When anger becomes sufficiently collective and organized, it generates political unrest. This is why political regimes struggle to legitimize or discredit certain forms of anger, a key to maintaining social order — and social movements are often reframed, and discredited, as emotional outbursts of anger (see Holmes, 2004 on feminist politics and anger). In contemporary China, Yang (2016) focuses on the forms of anger experienced by workers who were laid off by former state companies in Changping, a district of Beijing. Many became taxi drivers — a role in a service industry that requires emotional control. Three modes of displaying anger can be distinguished: *majie* (rant, literally cursing on streets, previously considered a feminine behaviour), *xiangpi ren* (silenced rage, highly pathologized and close to the Western burn out), and *nande hutu* ('muddledness as a more difficult kind of smartness'). Yang describes how laid-off workers and state-sponsored psychosocial workers use these angers differently, in a context where the Chinese state tends to regulate this anger — framing unrest as a crisis of masculinity rather than an economic issue — where Confucian and Daoist legacies influence collective perceptions, and where psychosocial workers ultimately attempt to domesticate this emotion.

Returning to the stress paradigm, these studies enable reassessment of the centrality of stress from a different angle: what is unveiled and concealed by the stress model? Or, in a more Marxist phrasing, who benefits from studying mental health in terms of stress, who is praised and who is discredited? The workers studied by Yang (2016) are certainly stressed. But summarizing their distress as stress may miss crucial details in understanding their situation. In contrast, considering anger, what it refers to politically and socially, who experiences it in what situation, facilitates a more contextually sensitive analysis of the relationship between feelings, distress and society. Anger, more than a cause or an outcome of mental disorders, can thus be used as a prism to comprehensively grasp certain social contexts potentially productive of mental disorders; as many other emotions.

Paranoia and the social organization of trust

Paranoia provides another example of this point. In the DSM-5 (2013), Paranoid Personality Disorder is the most explicit mention of paranoia, but other disorders, especially in schizophrenia, include the feeling that others want to hurt us, that a plot is organized against us, that people lie to manipulate us or that some messages are subconsciously or unconsciously directing our actions (which is a textbook definition of advertising or political communication). In its broadest sense, even negative thinking, prevalent in depression and other troubles, includes paranoid overtones.

In 1971, Cooper wrote: 'the therapist in working with people might far more often have to confirm the reality of paranoid fears than in any sense disconfirm or attempt to modify them' (p 11). This argument, as many anti-psychiatric arguments, has been accused of romanticizing mental illness. Still, this extract raises an important sociological question: who draws the line between fantasized persecution and real oppression? In his analysis of the changing nature of schizophrenia diagnoses in US psychiatric institutions in the twentieth century, Metzl (2010) notes that the 'paranoia' of many African American male patients was attributed by psychiatrists to a mental disorder: schizophrenia; and yet the content of these 'delusions' often portrayed conditions of racial injustice and inequality.

> 'It is a type of ruminating, loosely connected wishful thinking that certainly is not too factual. ... On one interview he talked about his color and he implied he had been subordinated because of that. ... He is keenly aware of his lack of social status and wealth. Yet he continues to hallucinate and he is often grandiose in his ruminations ... He denies that he is mentally ill.' (Psychiatrist's notes, 1950s, cited in Metzl, 2010, p 87)

Several sociological reflections emphasize the cumulating effects of social interactions, emerging out of social structures, in the development of paranoid delusions, especially among people holding disadvantaged statuses. Addressing the social sources of paranoia, Lemert (1962, p 14) stated that 'many paranoid persons properly realize that they are being isolated and excluded by concerted interaction, or that they are being manipulated'. This point was moved forward by Mirowsky and Ross (1983). To study paranoia sociologically, they reconceptualize it as 'belief in external control', which they assume to be more prevalent among lower social status individuals for whom feeling of (actual) powerlessness bolsters perceptions of a world controlled by potentially malevolent others; a finding that they substantiate with quantitative data collected in Texas, US, and Mexico.

Although the small literature on this topic mostly concentrates on disadvantaged people, we can also see paranoia as a sociological object being associated with a wider range of populations. Richards (1996) suggests that paranoid feeling might occur in expatriates during the process of adjustment to a new country: believing that locals organize themselves to make one's integration difficult. At a more societal level, it may be that material possession and comfort condition, by definition, the fear of loss. This leads Best (2001) to diagnose the 'paradox of paranoia' in Western societies: social progress, such as the advancement of medicine and hygiene, has perversely increased fears of collapse. Despite living in increasingly safer conditions, Westerners become more sensitive to the (smaller) risks of losing what they possess.

These initial reflections combine to suggest that paranoia, as a social emotion, is better understood in the frame of the *social organization of trust*, or how, in a given society some processes exist to credit or discredit, or how some institutions, discourses and actors produce unequal politics of credentials and surveillance. Fassin (2021) notes that while the COVID-19 pandemic of 2020 onwards confronted the general audience with fanciful 'conspiracy theories', these could be connected to *actual plots* exposed in previous decades: that of the tobacco and lead industries, or that of the US and UK governments pretending to have found weapons of mass destruction in Iraq. Paranoia, and conspiracies, can be understood as not merely individual 'weaknesses of reasoning', but as embedded in history – sometimes, they are a political sixth sense.

For paranoia to make sense in its psychiatric, individualized sense, it needs to occur in a peaceful society[10] whose most powerful actors – the state and private companies – are benevolent towards all citizens. Such a society does not currently exist, and thus the perception of safety and benevolence is only 'rational' for advantaged groups for whom, *indeed,* the state and private companies adopt well-intentioned and controlled initiatives. We have already evoked Harper's (2011) observations that both formal and informal surveillance affects certain groups more, from women to people of colour through the unemployed and the working class. CCTV, for example, is used for collective safety and law enforcement to protect people from various hazards; however, it is well understood that these policies do not impact all populations in the same way. Also, some state policies are based on paranoid logics, such as border policies that rely on the systematic suspicious of certain publics as dangerous, organized and ill-intentioned (Fassin, 2011b; Yildiz, 2016). This moral economy of trust does not randomly, or equally, permeate the social world.

To be clear, we do not suggest that psychiatrists always confound pathological paranoia with social domination, or that all forms of paranoia take root in actual plots. We suggest that we cannot understand individual paranoid symptoms without taking into consideration the whole social organization that revolves around surveillance, trust, credentials, and so forth, in a given society. This perspective blurs the boundaries between paranoia that is *unjustified* by the context, which the DSM identifies as symptom, and *justified* paranoia – actual plots, actual surveillance. In this frame, the identification of paranoid traits that appear under socially pathological forms cannot be separated from a broader questioning of the *social organization of trust*.

Conclusion

> Its bold, and perhaps most controversial, assumption is that everything that is represented by the components of the stress process – the social context, stressors, resources, and outcomes – can be conceived of as part of a more general, continual process by which people construct the meanings of life conditions in interaction with others. (McLeod, 2012, p 175)

Anger, paranoia, but also guilt, shame, boredom, sadness, excitement, apathy, obsession, mysticism, shyness, despair. The stress of being discriminated, being disappointed, losing one's house, being unable to buy a third one, feeling judged, observed, coming out, working until exhaustion, displaying toughness, staying polite in front of one's boss. There exists a multiplicity of activities and social processes in which stress holds a transcendent but limited role. Even the diversity of biological phenomena attached to stress – take the multiple vital and emotional phenomena tied to cortisol (Roberts and McWade, 2021) – suggests that the sheer diversity of human experience cannot be tackled *only* by differentiating several types of stress, nor by the isolation of 'stressors', 'buffers' and 'coping mechanisms'. The gaps we raise in this chapter will either require significant renewals, such as those proposed by McLeod (2012), Schieman (2019) and Simon (2020), or for other paradigms, more successful in accounting for the entanglement of emotional experiences, inequalities and agency in the genesis of mental health, to take over. The stress paradigm, once a path-breaking research perspective, might have reached its limits.

Coelho's fictional story of Veronika (1998) provided a counter-illustration, one which introduced our chapter on 'stress' and to which we now return. Veronika's desire to die is framed by Coelho as a response not to stress, but to boredom and predictability – a life planned out neatly, but one that lacks connection and meaning. A lack of stressful excitement in a context marked by classed and gendered expectations for Veronika's life, which is on a 'downhill trajectory'. Even once she took pills to end her life, Veronika is still bored. She uses what she thinks to be her remaining time writing a letter to a newspaper in which a previous article jokingly started with the question, 'Where is Slovenia?' – her country of origin. The letter explains where Slovenia is. As her mother later comments, maybe she wanted to die to 'put Slovenia on the map'. What if this seemingly funny detail of the story was an important one? At least, it hints at something important: how people try to make sense of their time, their life and their death. This underlines the vital roles of socially, culturally and historically situated meanings, further shaped by intersecting social roles and relations, in the production of stress – and other emotions. Much of what Veronika enrols in justifying her desire for death relates to an imagined future in a particular place and time.

Stress has a history of its own (Jackson, 2013) that partly helps to understand why it has been taken as a major driver of distress, especially in some fractions of the Anglo-European middle classes: this is the history of the production of people seeing themselves as potentially stressed, and seeking strategies to relieve their tensions. Rather than being a matter of biology, or even psychology, such a focus should be questioned as a moral economy in which social life is assessed through its potential to generate stress. This worldview underlies that inherently, some institutions and cultures provide sufficient means for people to make sense of their time, their emotions, their life and their death in a singularly fulfilling way: to be happy, *in the sense of* unstressed.

3

The Weight of Labels

Marge Piercy's novel *Woman on the Edge of Time* (1976) begins with Connie's psychiatric hospitalization for 'violent behaviour'. A working class, Latino woman in 1970s US, Connie was 'violent' indeed. She violently protected her niece against a pimp – hitting him with a bottle in an attempt to prevent her niece undergoing a forced abortion. Living in a threatening neighbourhood, she might have used violence in other situations, or become used to it. But decontextualized 'violence' appears inadmissible, pathological, morally reprehensible. In this story, mental health professionals decontextualize Connie's actions, making them illegitimate, the sign of an individual flaw, and this had terrible outcomes. Tragically, Connie finds herself locked up and dispossessed from the custody of her child. But in the hospital, a ray of hope shines in the form of Luciente's visits. Luciente introduces Connie into a bright future, a fulfilling, utopian social organization that Connie can eventually explore by herself, meeting its members, discovering how their community overcame the plagues of capitalism, individualism and sexism. Whether these visits are imaginary or real is another question.

In the society Connie discovers, words implement change. A significant one is 'per'. Per, the first three letters of 'person', is used instead of 'he' or 'she', both as an outcome and catalyst of the shifting gender relations that drove this future world out of masculine domination: people are referred to as persons, not as sexes. As such, some parts of this story critique how institutions categorize behaviours in a way that minimizes their social context, especially for those who, like Connie, do not have the means to resist. Further, *Woman on the Edge of Time* raises reflections on the power carried by categorizations. What does it mean to be 'violent'? What does it mean to be called 'he', 'she' – 'per'? Categories are hinges between realities and their perception. As such, because people live through how they name things, labelling mechanisms have both conservative and transformative potential: they draw a space of possibilities.

This is why, in sociology, the processes through which 'troubles', 'disorders' or 'diseases' are given names, represented and made official by some institutions, constitute a major research focus (Jutel, 2009). Social scientists refer to these names as labels, categories, diagnoses or even discourses, depending on the theoretical traditions in which they are embedded. These concepts highlight that our experience and how we interpret its various disruptions rely on socially and historically variable categories. Mental disorders are worded, interpreted in context, and these idioms can and do change. Still, their names do not lightly mirror the cultures in which they appear, as underneath any category, some institutional actors likely contributed to the production and application of these labels. In doing so, institutions inevitably colour these never-neutral labels with their worldviews – the medical classifications (the Diagnostic and Statistical Manual of Mental Disorders and the International Classification of Diseases) released by the American Psychiatric Association and the World Health Organization are widely studied for this reason. Classifications have deep impact: people integrate psychiatric categories into their semantic repertoire to make sense of their problems, while professionals employ them as authoritative designations, with far reaching effects on the lives of those who are labelled. Finally, one cannot live outside categorizations – if only to reject them – and much research accounts for this phenomenon, from the most descriptive options, where labels qualify pre-existing disorders, to more radical approaches, where labels create the disorders to which they give a name.

In short, *categories have a generative power*. But what power exactly? What is the relationship between labels and the realities they qualify? What is the weight of labels?

This chapter begins in the 1960s, when social theory shifted in its understanding of categorization processes. We exemplify this 'great reversal' with two figures of that time. While the labelling theory of mental illness was developed by Thomas Scheff from the warm suburbs of Santa Barbara, Michel Foucault proposed, from the coldest Parisian streets, an epistemological view of madness standing at the core of the Western self. Both approaches achieved immense academic and public traction. Although Scheff and Foucault situated the production of mental health within a wider social landscape populated with overlapping norms, institutions, knowledges and power, most subsequent approaches took less speculative and therefore narrower lenses, examining labelling processes and devices through medicalization, daily categorizations and stigma. After reviewing these trends, we outline some avenues for contemporary research, tentatively preserving the best of both worlds, tying the empirical study of labelling processes with broader reflections on their sociocultural implication. This will drive us to spotlight three areas of exploration: the socio-political arrangements at the core of label production; the performativity of categories; and the 'function' of labels in social organization.

Great reversals

This idea that labels vary between and within societies was certainly not new in the 1960s. Since the nineteenth century, anthropologists observed that all around the world, different peoples have different ways of understanding health and illness (Kaiser and Kohrt, 2019); social historians and psychiatrists themselves documented the transformation of categories over time (Bromberg, 1942); and some sociologists, such as Parsons (1951), had already pioneered studies of diseases taken as deviances expressing contingent social norms. Scheff and Foucault represent a turn in this history. Coming from dramatically different theoretical backgrounds, along with others such as Goffman,[1] they embodied the renewal of approaches to categorization in the study of mental health. Each promoted the idea that labels contribute to the realities they designate, and that underneath those categories lies a whole symbolic world in which madness only represents a cog. We will emphasize the *performative ontology* fuelling both of these influential benchmarks in sociological thought.

The labelling theories of mental illness

A basic formulation of labelling can be summarized as such: a trouble occurs, and a label is used to define its nature [trouble → label]. For instance, someone who experiences a long-lasting feeling of sadness may go to see a professional and receive a diagnosis of depression. In this frame, the label does nothing more than characterize the trouble, giving it a name, which helps the concerned persons to mobilize pre-existing knowledge on this disorder and seek treatment. Labelling *theory* reverses this formulation: instead of considering that *labels label some already-present reality*, it asserts that *labels produce the reality they label* [label → trouble]. When someone is diagnosed with depression, this influences the course of their disorder, but more essentially, the very existence of the label 'depression' has created – beforehand – a series of representations and activities that shapes the way in which people experience and interpret the associated emotions in a given society.

Although this framework had already surfaced in earlier studies (Lemert, 1951; Becker, 1963), Scheff's book *Being Mentally Ill* (1966) formalized labelling theory for mental illness, in close relation to the sociology of deviance and the anti-psychiatric movement. Its starting point is that most individuals internalize norms throughout their life. From early childhood, they are provided with notions encouraging them to separate so-called transgressions from so-called normal behaviours; they learn to 'know', rather intuitively, what behaviours are appropriate or not. If someone steals your jacket, they are a 'thief' and should be apprehended by the police. If a high school student cheats at an exam, they are a 'cheater' and may be send to the headteacher. Transgression, categorization, institutionalization. However, some rules are much more tacit. Some transgressions are not written anywhere. They are *felt*, transgressive because they disturb taken-for-granted expectations. There is no law prohibiting hallucinations; however, when someone hallucinates, this may unsettle those around them, and themselves. No rulebook bans mood changes too, but similarly, such changes might be problematic to the person and others. Scheff was clear that most *residual transgressions* are normalized, tolerated as transient, meaningless eccentricities. Only some endure and are judged too disruptive. Only at this point might they trigger a progressive qualification of the individual, under a label of mental illness. Only then, individuals experiencing repeated hallucinations or drastic mood changes are – because people around them previously internalized certain representations of madness and because specialized institutions have traced ideal-typical recovery trajectories for these disturbances – eventually diagnosed, here with schizophrenia or bipolar disorders.[2]

Labelling theory has left an immense legacy, becoming one of the pillars of social constructionism in mental health research (see Bowers, 1998; Rogers and Pilgrim, 2014), along with Goffman's *Asylum* (1961) and *Stigma* (1963), that at the same moment drew attention to how 'spoilt identities' produced by psychiatric institutions and everyday stigmatization could turn the lives of people deemed crazy upside down. *Being Mentally Ill* aroused passionate controversy, both through attempts to test it (Rosenhan, 1973) and to detract from it (Davis, 1972). Disagreements crystallized in the *American Sociological Review* of the mid-1970s (Scheff, 1974, 1975; Gove, 1975, 1976). Gove reproached labelling theory for being based on empirically unverifiable concepts such as 'internalized social control'. Thoits (1985) argued that Scheff's model was most relevant to severe disorders like chronic schizophrenia, while Link (et al, 1989) suggested it was not able to encompass diseases for which 'organic causes' are suspected. Goldstein (1979, pp 387–391) raised that it often draws attention to instances of ambiguous deviance where bureaucratic biases obviously orient the labelling of a disorder.

In view of these criticisms, it is worth insisting on Scheff's original message. Labelling theory has often been misinterpreted, Pollner (1978) explains, due to the confusion between its 'mundane version', where the community is understood as an umpire in which professionals give right or wrong labels to people, whereas in its sociological 'constitutive version', community is the inventor of the game. In other words, labelling processes do not only involve naming a set of symptoms (and even less in a good or bad way). They are productive social forces setting up the *conditions of possibility* for mental disorders. This is why methodological critiques of labelling theory should be treated cautiously. Maybe this theory is not conducive to being converted into falsifiable hypotheses.[3] As Goldstein (1979) notes, labelling theory cannot be 'evidenced', but some of its aspects can be discussed with empirical data (Sherlock and Kielich, 1991). In its broadest interpretation, this theory encourages study of how labels contribute to building the symbolic worlds we inhabit, where certain labels assign people exhibiting 'disturbing' behaviours to the margins.

This ocean of criticisms, of which we merely report the highest waves, led to interesting developments. Thoits (1985) draws attention to self-labelling. Especially with the least severe disorders, she observed that individuals tend to label themselves *before* being labelled by others. Faced with an emotional or behavioural deviance, they firstly suspect themselves of having some mental health problem, before consulting professionals. Professionals may then confirm or invalidate the would-be-patient's worry. The diagnosis thus 'reassures' patients; it helps them to put a name on a previously unidentified problem. On their side, Link and colleagues (1989) developed a 'modified labelling theory', in which labelling facilitates relapses but cannot, as Scheff claimed, generate the disease in the first place. They also insist on the importance of anticipated stigma: the simple – but often true – belief that social rejection can follow problems deemed 'psychiatric' have a decisive influence on mental health trajectories. In sum, both Thoits and Link 'softened' the initial theory of labelling, mirroring changes in US psychiatry, which was becoming less coercive than two decades earlier, and in the sociology of mental health, which was becoming less radically critical of psychiatry.

A related area of work can be identified in Emerson and Messinger's (1977; Emerson, 2015) 'micro-politics of trouble'. Building on the Goffmanian framework in which social life is vulnerable, constantly endangered by small 'troubles', they note that, when such troubles become more problematic and recurrent, worried persons (either the individual themselves or their relatives) may ask for advice from those around them, either people they already know or professional specialists. Emerson and Messinger argue that it is *through* this help-seeking process, through being exposed to words and categories aimed at making sense of their difficulties, that people acquire a certain understanding of their trouble, shaping how the trouble is later defined, experienced and potentially resolved.

In comparison with labelling theory, the 'micro-politics of trouble' offers a more methodologically approachable take on labelling processes, through networks of acquaintances and relations with diverse persons and institutions. For example, it allows differentiation of the protagonists at play between those who perform 'intrinsic remedies' (within existing relations, such as support from relatives already known by the troubled person before troubles started) and 'third parties,' between non-professional, generalist and specialized professionals. Furthermore, this model encourages consideration of not-yet-labelled troubles, *prior to* labelling, which reveals an important trend in current research: most sociologists of mental health examine already-labelled troubles, pre-selecting those who fall into the realm of psychiatry and psychology, which is a restricted, slightly teleological, way of demonstrating the social construction of mental disorders.

Madness, power and knowledge

In another context, inspired by Canguihlem's (1943) reflections on the normal and the pathological, which shows the social and scientific articulations surrounding the designation of the pathological in societies, Foucault took a step further. Throughout *History of Madness* (1961) and *The Birth of the Clinic* (1963), he initiated a path-breaking perspective whereby rationality and madness, in the last centuries, became two sides of the same coin. This shift occurred through institutional and social arrangements among which psychiatry (first materialized by confinement structures) played a key role. According to Foucault, the historical development of medical knowledge and practice, rather than unveiling some distinction between the normal and the pathological, resulted in the formation of a discursive space where the 'mad' are materially and symbolically excluded from mainstream society; but in so doing, perhaps counter-intuitively, such marginalization bolstered the establishment of bourgeois morality, science and the progress of reason.

The theoretical framework underlying these intuitions was later elaborated with *The Order of Things* (1966) and *The Archaeology of Knowledge* (1969), where Foucault dissected the set of tacit assumptions that make knowledge possible – *episteme*. Like a cultural historian, he analysed the semantic associations, representations, and ways of conceptualizing the truth typical to each *episteme*. Within these reflections, madness appears as one of these discursive formations that organize our way of seeing the world, insofar as psychiatry and its tools generated an 'articulated space of possible descriptions' (Foucault, 1969, p 62). Henceforth, the figure of madness does not stand at the margins of our social world, but represents a constitutive part of its discursive landscape and government devices.

Armstrong (1997, p 67) points out that a pivotal subtext transcends the *Birth of the Clinic*: 'the emergence of the individual'. It is true that the spread in Western societies of observation and control devices, such as the hospital, raises questions about what type of subject could emerge in such a context. This idea was further elaborated in *Discipline and Punish* (1975) and the *History of Sexuality* (1976), where Foucault drifts away from the 'legal approach' that conceives power as the rules that *restrict* people's behaviours and ideas. Famously inquiring into British Victorian society and the French monarchy, he demonstrates that power encompasses a *generative* dimension in social life, as the design of restrictions ultimately lead practices, discourses and desires to emerge. By extension, institutions of social control (police, psychiatry, and so on) provide societies with modes of subjectivation, that is, ways of becoming subjects. A key aspect of Foucault's arguments was that a Western shift from political systems where visceral public punishment enacted sovereign rule to more diffuse and 'positive' types of governmentality did not necessarily imply more freedom or constraint, but rather different methods of regulating 'desiring selves'. In this picture, much in the same way 'homosexuality' as a category and identity was elaborated through its prohibition, 'madness' characterizes the nascent type of individuals emerging in the classical era through a certain form of 'rational' governmentality.

How might we draw on this legacy today? Some authors have successfully extended Foucault's approach regarding the status of medicine and illness in contemporary societies. Castel et al (1982; see also Castel, 1988) observed that the traditional management of madness through psychiatry and hospitals was progressively reconfigured as a decentralized network of expertise, policies and professionals of all kinds, who concentrate on the minimization of risks and the treatment of vulnerabilities; a 'post-disciplinary' order that reconfigures how psychiatry and psychology 'manage the social'. In the same vein, Armstrong (1995) heralded the rise of *surveillance medicine*, which, following the models of 'bedside medicine' and 'hospital medicine' identified by Foucault, displays salient features: medicine does not only refer to professionals who are in charge of curing illnesses anymore, but of anticipating them in monitoring risks, including among healthy people, beyond the wall of institutions, in the community. To summarize, these works suggest that psy-institutions have moved from preserving 'normal' society from 'madness' to managing omnipresent threats to 'health'. These observations fit well with the later explosion of mental health-related discourses, and the 'mental health crisis'.[4]

Another extension of the Foucauldian legacy explores contemporary modes of governmentality and the making of selves. Rose (1990, 1996, 2018) epitomizes this orientation as he demonstrates how the development of psychiatry, psychology and other 'psy-professions', contributed to a vision of the 'self' that transformed how individuals are shaped and governed by institutions. Rose's work describes discourses signalling the rise of a reflective, psychologized, neoliberal self that ultimately makes 'calculable minds and manageable individuals' (Rose, 1988). Fassin similarly furthered Foucault's approach to governmentality. To him, mental health-related issues are aspects of contemporary moral economies, which can be tracked through from the development of community organizations promoting 'listening' as a soft form of governance, especially targeting the working class (Fassin, 2004), to the pervasiveness of the concept of trauma and the status of 'victim' on a global scale (Fassin and Rechtman, 2009). Fassin observes the development of both a 'compassionate ethos' and of the 'humanitarian reason' (Fassin, 2011c): the suffering of others and its recognition became a prism through which political intervention is thought and legitimized. Both Fassin and Rose argue that the shifts occurring in how mental health and illness are understood, experienced and responded to, are entangled with changing modes of governmentality and associated discursive formations – the diffusion of psy-discourses, neoliberal selves, the use of 'listening' institutions, and suffering as a motor of political action.

Foucault's approach has also been qualified as 'revisionist' by some historians such as Scull (1989, 2019). Indeed, Foucault revised a classical 'progress' narrative of psychiatric history made of upward steps accompanying the progress of science. However, his 'revision' still embraces history as a progressive albeit deceptive shift from coercion to moral treatment; and Scull points out several inaccuracies in Foucault's archival research. To be sure, the 'Foucault industry' (Scull, 2019, p 27) should not be taken as a historical reference – it has also been deemed quite abstract (Hacking, 2004). Its interest lies in the genealogical approach that merged two separate aims: revisiting history with present questions, and legitimizing discourse analysis as a way of unveiling the social construction of reality. While the intricacies of this approach – and the difficulty of clarity due to the complexity of Foucault's writing – cannot be discussed in this book as they do not explicitly attend to the explanation of mental disorders, let us retain a somewhat generic recommendation: there is a co-occurring generative process tying together discourses, practices, selves, knowledges and governmentality.

Into the politics of categorization

Both Scheff and Foucault (1) approached representations of 'madness' as generated by and generative of a society's core normative structure, (2) conceptualized labels not as mere categories only qualifying forms of mental disorders but parts of normative knowledges *productive* of these disorders, and (3) suggested studying these processes empirically without excluding more theoretical reflections on what they mean to societies as a whole. They invited us to pay attention to how labels are created, what they mean in social life, what they tell us about the societies we live in, how they are used and resisted, with what consequences, in what institutions, with what expertise. These propositions were welcomed as unforgettable lessons for many sociologists of mental health. From now on, studying how mental disorders 'appear' involves exploring the productive dimension of the associated categories, as well as the institutions and knowledge systems in which they take place.

Pilgrim (2007) contends that three main epistemological positions can be found regarding diagnosis, a view that can be extended to mental health categories at large. *Medical naturalism*, sometimes also called realism, considers that diagnoses label things that already exist in the nature. This is the stereotypical biomedical position. In opposition, *radical constructivism* sees diagnoses as the subjective product of human activity, and therefore the problems they label do not 'really' exist. *Critical realism*, Pilgrim advances, bridges these two positions in considering that mental disorders both exist and are produced by human activity; this 'third way' resembles Hacking's (1995b, 1999) *dynamic nominalism* and his notion of 'looping effect'. An agenda is set: social perspectives do not show that mental disorders do not exist. Rather, they study the articulation between categories and the realities they help to construct. What people say, the categories they use, how they frame the world dramatically shapes their – symbolic and material – realities. But how?

This calls for consideration of the *politics of categorization*. From the 1980s onwards, three related research axes developed in the sociology of mental health: the study of how labels are made and legitimized, of how they are negotiated in specific settings, and of their consequences on people and societies. We will review these axes, taking stock of what they bring to our understanding of the sociogenesis of mental disorders.

How labels acquire legitimacy: medicalization processes

How are mental health categories created, legitimized, and diffused? What leads some human behaviours and emotions to be attached to a label that signals their belonging to the realm of the pathological?

In the social sciences, these questions have been predominantly tackled through the concept of *medicalization*: the process by which a problem is framed as a medical condition, thus becoming the object of medical study, diagnosis, prevention, and treatment (Conrad and Schneider, 1980; Busfield, 2017). Building on seminal studies (Pitts, 1968; Freidson, 1970; Zola, 1972), Conrad and Schneider (1980) authored its now mainstream definition. Since then, medicalization has become an umbrella term for research projects that monitor the historical evolution of physical and mental health conditions. Examples include attention deficit hyperactivity disorder (ADHD; Conrad and Potter, 2000), shyness through social phobia, social anxiety disorder and avoidant personality disorder (Scott, 2006), self-harm (Ekman, 2016) and various issues surrounding sexuality (Flore, 2020). But how can medicalization help us understand the emergence of mental disorders? What makes medicalization happen in the first place?

Many works present medicalization as resulting from the activities of influential actors who act out of professional prestige and material interests.[5] In this reasoning, the quest of professional influence leads some actors to invest time, money and energy in the medicalization of an extending range of behaviours and emotions.

Originally, Conrad and Schneider (1980) positioned the empowerment of the medical profession over the twentieth century as a major factor in the increase of medicalization processes in Western societies. Since the 1960s and 1970s, medical authority, social movements, and competition between professionals combine in this process (Conrad, 2007, p 9). Following this path, most studies focus on how a disorder becomes institutionalized by a medical authority – often the American Psychiatric Association – supported by pharmaceutical companies and/or other interest groups, which fosters the popularity of a category that individuals can adopt as their own (Scott, 1990, about PTSD; Horwitz, 2011, and Shorter, 2013 about depression; Nadesan, 2005, about autism; Schnittker, 2020, about the DSM).

This approach was subsequently extended in view of the considerable power held by pharmaceutical industries. Some scholars develop concepts such as 'biomedicalization' (Clarke et al, 2003), 'pharmaceuticalization' (Abraham, 2010; Collin and David, 2016) or even 'disease mongering' (Moyinhan et al, 2002). This relates to the marketization of medicine, especially in the US, where the focus has shifted from the 'whole body' and 'body as parts' to the 'molecular body', including DNA, hormonal focus or the micromanagement of blood sugar (Rose, 2007).

Another way to understand medicalization consists of asking why, in a given context, certain categories 'work', or resonate with, some traits of the culture in which they develop. In this reasoning, the spotlight is less focused on the activities of powerful actors, attending more to broader cultural transformations on which medicalization processes (and individual motivations to medicalize) are reliant.

For instance, Barbee et al (2018, p 12) link the medicalization of sleeplessness to American neoliberalism characterized by 'enhancement culture, commodification of health, and a "productivity imperative"', while Maturo and Moretti (2018) argue that capitalism-based anxiety helps to explain the success of phone applications that medicalize everyday life – here medicalization being taken in its broadest sense. Several cultural dimensions have also been evoked to explain the popularity of sex addiction, a controversial category included in the DSM from 1987 to 1994 (or 2013, if we consider its 'equivalent', hypersexuality): intimacy issues in post-industrial societies (Keane, 2004), moral panic in the HIV/AIDS era, the backlash of the 1960s 'sexual emancipation' (Reay et al, 2015; Irvine, 1995), the stabilization of pornography as a genre and the extension of the addiction concept (Taylor, 2019).

A key issue for the medicalization literature soon revolved around its *scale of analysis*. Medicalization was long approached as a macro-social phenomenon; however, not only can notable variations be observed 'on the ground', sometimes contradicting macro-social trends (Halfmann, 2011), but also both patients and professionals can have agency (Valentine, 2010) and therefore can resist this process (Roy et al, 2019; Nelson, 2019; Whooley, 2010). If the medical conceptions legitimized in classifications such as the DSM or ICD are understood and enacted in diverse ways, what are the implications of investigating these classifications? In addition, some disorders now grow outside the medical realm – sex addiction being an example – and thus question the centrality of the medical apparatus in the production of mental health categories. Are we moving from medicalization to *legitimation*, a term Friberg (2009) uses to understand the history of 'burn out', a category not present in the DSM? How can we comprehensively explore the complex and changing socio-political arrangements that 'generate' disorders through medicalization?

Labels in everyday life: local settings and agency

Local settings influence the way in which labels are negotiated, which influences how mental disorders take shape in people's lives.

Inspired by microsociology and ethnography, many scholars have turned the grand theories previously outlined into methodological examinations of how labelling occurs in practice. This trend has been nurtured by the rising sociology of diagnosis, taken as an interactive and iterative process that has productive effects on the health problems thus designated (Blaxter, 1978; Brown, 1995; Jutel, 2009; McGann et al, 2011; Jutel and Nettleton, 2011), leading researchers to focus on different facets of the labelling process.

Labelling entails interactions in which some complaints are identified, categorized and narrated. For instance, 'being sad and tired', or 'thinking too much', might be reframed as 'depression' or 'anxiety disorder' *in interaction*. This transformative operation has been detailed in different manners. O'Reilly et al (2020) present mental health assessments as 'rhetorical cases' and Maynard and Turowetz (2019) as 'narrative procedures'. These operations through which professionals transform their clients' words into clinical idioms are sometimes called 're-phrasing' (Bonnin, 2017), 'reformulation' (LeVine and Matsuda, 2003) or 'resignification' (Mora-Rios et al, 2016). Note that these formulations are not necessarily communicated to the patient (see Moran and Karnieli-Miller, 2014, about diagnosis disclosure). These works imply that the situational and semantic reframing of complaints play a significant role in the experience of the disorder.

Labelling reflects the professional organization prevailing in a given institutional setting, and in a given geographical area. Barrett's (1996) classical study of schizophrenia in an Australian psychiatric ward demonstrated how each professional advanced their own lens to analyse the patients' issues, producing oral and written reports underscoring the dimensions their professional socialization led them to see, building a 'case', that is, the composite, clinical and likely performative depiction of a patient. A 'case' mirrors a division of labour, where the biomedical perspective, written about by the psychiatrist, is deemed the deepest layer of a patient's personality, while social environment, written about by the social worker, appears as an 'external', less important layer.

In contrast, Bonnin (2020) describes an Argentinian facility where the key professional divide is between proponents of psychiatric biomedicine and that of psychoanalysis, each with significantly different worldviews on therapeutic options and the very conception of mental health. This opposition, articulated through hospital bureaucracy, generates tensions in the interactions between professionals and patients (who assume that all the hospital staff follow the medical model). In short, labelling processes – that largely determine the course of disorders – are contingent on the organization of work, itself the result of contextual and institutional structures.

Labels are also affixed through interactions that include non-professionals. In particular, families play a significant role in the social framing of troubles. Even in diagnostic encounters, relatives are often present: what is their influence on diagnosis itself? Chua (2012) observes that in South India, symptoms are formulated primarily as accusations among members of the family for not complying with traditional enactments of domesticity and kinship. Whether families structure the diagnosis process, particularly in Kerala, could be discussed, but similar features have been noted, especially when the troubled person is a child or teenager, in many other contexts such as the US (Carpenter-Song, 2009; Francis, 2015) or in France (Blum, Minoc and Weber, 2015). However, the influence of non-professionals in labelling and diagnosis processes still tends to be downplayed in the literature.

Once diagnosed, or at least exposed to a mental health category, people use this potential frame to reassess their life and problems, eventually modifying their self-conception. Many recent studies inquire into this aspect, among adolescents (Moses, 2009), offenders (Dixon, 2015), hospitalized women (Pope, 2015) or veterans (Spoont et al, 2009). For example, Kokanovic et al (2013) explore how people diagnosed with depression in Australia integrate this diagnosis into their life story. Some appropriate 'depression' as a tool to elaborate the narrative they have of themselves, such as in introducing new explanatory elements of their current state. Some accept, refuse or reduce the medication they are prescribed, moving 'inside and outside a medicalised discourse' (Kokanovic et al, 2013, p 384).

Another example is provided by Tran (2017), who analyses how Vietnamese psychiatrists interpret declarations of 'worry' among their patients through the prism of 'generalized anxiety disorder' while patients favour the older medical term, 'neurasthenia', which better echoes a legitimate sense of moral obligation underlying their emotions, thus closer to their self-definition. In a nutshell, labelling processes represent and interact with potentially transformative identity reconfigurations.

Some studies emphasize greater balance between the 'positive' and 'negative' effects of labelling, noting that diagnosis can *help* renegotiate one's identity (Fernandez et al, 2014), trigger a 'positive feeling' (Killingsworth et al, 2010), or even reinforce biographical cohesion (Skovbo Rasmussen et al, 2020). In the case of autism in the US, Tan (2018) goes as far as writing that diagnosis can constitute a 'biographical illumination', 'a transformed conceptualization of self and identity that is facilitated by but extends beyond medical meaning, enriching personal biography and social relationships' (p 164). Johnson (2019) shows that transgender people in the US develop an ambivalent relation to the 'gender dysphoria' diagnostic category, sometimes rejecting it for improperly medicalizing their situation, while strategically using medical arguments to justify their need for hormone treatments or in mundane exchanges. As one participant explains: 'it helps folks to be able to look at something and say, "oh, medically speaking … oh, you were born that way"' (Johnson, 2019, p 526). In sum, diagnoses do not only carry tragedies, they can also contribute to the – potentially positive – development of selves, which ultimately raises questions about the relations between the emergence of certain mental disorders and perceived needs for personal/social change.

By extension, people do not 'receive' medical expertise as passive subjects: this drives us to the topic of resistance. There is quite a fundamental disconnection between those who interpret resistance as a form of empowerment in the face of psychiatric domination (for instance, Bonnin, 2020) and those, closer to public health, who understand the same issue in terms of lack of compliance (see Reynolds et al, 2020). This topic has acquired particular significance since the 1990s, with online spaces enabling public discussion of mental health categories without any professional supervision. Ethnographies of digital communities (Giles and Newbold, 2011; Giles, 2014), as well as studies of the media (Ross Arguedas, 2020) and advocacy groups (Chamak, 2008), unveil arenas of relative autonomy from medical discourses. Digital spaces arguably foster the creation of a discrepancy between 'official' knowledges and lay knowledges (see Cresswell, 2005, about self-harm; Nettleton et al, 2005), and new ways of managing the visibility of mental health issues (Hendry, 2017).

But professionals can also express some distance towards some aspects of their labelling activities. On the one hand, diagnostic categories themselves are far from uncontested, as studies of medicalization demonstrate. 'Borderline personality disorders' is a case in point (Koehne et al, 2013; Sulzer, 2015) and psychiatry remains a realm of manifold doubts (Whooley, 2019), which generates issues worded as contradiction (Hayes et al, 2021), ambiguity (Hollin and Pilnick, 2018) or uncertainty (Lane, 2020; Pickersgill, 2020; Adeponle et al, 2015; Rafalovich, 2005). On the other hand, professionals do not mechanically endorse the 'mainstream' perspectives they are socialized in. They can doubt whether these perspectives apply to their particular context, as Kitanaka (2008) describes with Japanese psychiatrists who ambivalently adopted the Western notion of pathological suicide, caught between global psychiatry and the traditional notion of free-will based suicide, 'suicide of resolve'. Or they can preserve more or less systematic margins of resistance in clinical settings (Lane, 2020; Nelson, 2019; Whooley, 2010).

To conclude, there is a steady interest in the study of how labels, and especially diagnoses, are performed in situated contexts. Such interest has led to important contributions in the sociology of mental health, highlighting that diagnoses do not directly flow from symptoms, nor are they merely placed over subjects by psychiatric influence: interactions and settings are thick filters where discourses circulate, make sense, are altered, resisted and realized; interactions are where mental illnesses, their experience and understanding are partly elaborated. These perspectives further develop our understanding of the role of labels in the social genesis of mental disorders: if categorization shapes troubles, and if categorization depends on situations, then we must consider the weight of local particularities. This perspective has been increasingly developed, in recent literature, through the notion of stigma.

Stigma, or the shift towards consequences

From the 1990s onward, research on *stigma* thrived in sociology, social psychology and psychology, shifting the focus away from causes to consequences – a trend later accompanied by the development of disability studies. Stigma research situates *reactions* to mental disorders at the core of a spiral of negative outcomes that affects the life of concerned people, from amplifying their distress to reducing their recovery chances. A consensus exists around this idea: stigmatizing mental illness fosters mental illness.

Something of a victim of its own success, stigma became an ambiguous, multi-faceted concept (Livingston and Boyd, 2010). Goffman's (1963) original definition has been amply taken up, from critical theory to quantitative psychology, with qualitative or experimental methods. It has been applied to multiple situations from that of exotic dancers to people suffering from leprosy (Link and Phelan, 2001: pp 363–364). It has been made compatible with the language of public policies (Carter et al, 2014). Beyond its original formulation as a social process (Wallace, 2012), stigma now designates numerous layers and scales of negative social reactions[6] (Manago, 2015), often enlarged to any activity and thought that convey disapproval and trigger discomfort, such as 'patronizing attitudes' (Dinos et al, 2004).

Stigma studies often rely on quantitative surveys evaluating the prevalence, form and effect of stigma either in general populations, among stigmatized people or among potential stigmatizers (Pescosolido, 2013; Sadler et al, 2012; Wright et al, 2011). Experiments and vignette methods assess how public stereotypes affect attitudes towards people with mental illnesses (Kroska et al, 2014; McGinty et al, 2015; Pescosolido et al, 2019). Increasingly, qualitative studies draw attention to the experience of stigma (Lee et al, 2006; Moses, 2010).

Across these studies, a number of coherent findings can be identified.

Levels of stigmatization remain very high in most societies, even when institutions and policies promote tolerance (Link and Phelan, 2001), while types of stigma vary depending on cultures and disorders (Knifton, 2012).

Stigma is understood as standing at the centre of a downward spiral where people suffering from mental health problems, stigmatized, become more affected by their problems (Marcussen et al, 2019), through lower self-esteem (Marcussen et al, 2019), lower help-seeking and access to services (Prior, 2012; Wright et al, 2011), lower recognition of the problem in family (Villatoro et al, 2018b), lower employment, less social relations, and more difficulties recovering or managing symptoms (Hayward and Bright, 1997; Link and Phelan, 2001). 'Positive' effects are sometimes noted, such as strengthening strong ties (while damaging peripheral ties, as in Perry, 2011) and being 'energized' (Corrigan and Watson, 2002).

Stigma has been shown to operate at several levels, each being characterized by a wide vocabulary: (a) intrapersonal or internalized; (b) interpersonal or meso-social; and (c) structural or macro-social (Livingston and Boyd, 2010; Manago, 2015; Woodgate et al, 2020). Schulze and Angermeyer (2003) distinguish between stigma in interpersonal interaction, structural discrimination, public images of mental illness and access to social roles.

Within everyday life, stigma takes multiple forms, from devaluation or avoidance to rejection and social control (Perry et al, 2020; Hinshaw, 2007, Chapter 6) and can come from different sources, from health professionals (Wallace, 2012; Taguibao and Rosenheck, 2021) to advertising (Payton and Thoits, 2011; Smardon, 2008). Stigma combines with other social disadvantages and discriminations, for instance among minorities (Perales and Todd, 2018; Qi and Wu, 2018), associated with serological status (Miller et al, 2016; Simbayi et al, 2007) or sanctioning social position (Wang et al, 2010).

Stigma extends to family members (Larson and Corrigan, 2008; Gray, 2002; Tzeng and Lipson, 2004; Song et al, 2018; Krupchanka et al, 2018). and to mental health professionals (Verhaeghe and Bracke, 2012 talk about 'associative stigma'). Even politicians might fear being associated with 'madness' in working on related policies (Sartorius, 2007).

People can *resist stigma*, in refusing stigmatization or refusing to stigmatize (Thoits and Link, 2016; Jenkins and Carpenter-Song, 2008; Whitley and Campbell, 2014). Resistance sometimes includes concealment strategies (Quinn et al, 2017) and the help of online communities (Yeshua-Katz, 2015). A question remains: can resistance really mitigate the consequences of stigma (Camp et al, 2002), especially when stigma is deeply embedded in structural and cultural processes (Tyler, 2020)?

The main explanation of stigma present in the literature is that *stigma results from misconceptions and detrimental stereotypes*. This argument is apparent in studies that seek to measure the efficacy of stigma reduction campaigns or 'mental health literacy' initiatives (Evans-Lacko, 2014; Kohrt et al, 2020; Sercu and Bracke, 2017; Vyncke and Van Gorp, 2020). Each of these starts from the premise that if people only knew more about a condition this would lead them to think and behave in less stigmatizing ways. However, many doubts remain, including who should be targeted by these campaigns – stigmatized publics, potential 'stigmatizers' or the general population (Corrigan and Fong, 2014)?

A variation of this argument is attribution theory, according to which a major factor in stigmatization is assumptions about culpability, where those with mental illnesses are understood as somehow at fault, bringing their troubles upon themselves. This theory has been challenged by studies which find that stigmatizing attitudes towards mental illness (or addiction) generally *do not* appear to be lessened when people also hold understandings of these as being biologically or more specifically genetically caused (Phelan, 2005; Meurk et al, 2014; Andersson and Harkness, 2018). Thus, stigma relating to mental illness remains even if individuals are not deemed responsible.

Although stigma studies have a prominent position in the social sciences, and particularly with regard to mental illness, their main challenge today is to overcome the social psychological bias which tends to consider 'stigma' as a universal trend, comparable and neutral. People do not stigmatize on a blank page; they live in an already stratified world where stigma is only the tip of the iceberg. We cannot cut stigmatizing behaviours off from the historical processes that generate them and enable their existence in the first place, such as cultural imperialism and marginalization (Bonnington and Rose, 2014; Tyler, 2020). Similarly, information campaigns might change how people perceive certain disorders and, ideally, trigger more acceptance towards those experiencing these disorders, for instance accepting them as co-workers or friends. However, the classification of behaviours and emotions in terms of mental health can itself be seen as a form of stigmatization or, rather, mental health stigma might be a superficial problem 'covering' various other inequalities and justifying the very constraining norms through which our emotional and behavioural differences are framed (Tyler 2020; Tyler and Slater, 2018).

In sum, stigma cannot be viewed only as an 'outcome' of mental illness. Mental health categories, the processes through which they form and the reactions they evoke in others cannot be isolated from their sociohistorical origins. Hence we invite, in agreement with Fraser et al (2017), on addiction, a view of stigma as a 'contingent biopolitically performative process' (p 192) – unstable and subject to contestation, rather than inherent to particular mental health experiences and categories. We continue to build on this key insight in the next section.

Back to the generative power of labelling

Mental health research addressing labelling processes has undergone major transformations since the 1960s. While Foucault and Scheff's seminal reflections dealt with the holistic mechanisms underlying mental health categorizations – from childhood socialization to governmentality – most contemporary works have *specialized*. This specialization has enabled an unparalleled degree of methodological sophistication, both in qualitative and quantitative approaches. Additionally, contemporary research has moved away from the slippery slope of *causality*, either privileging 'testable' hypotheses on the consequences of labelling practices, or, when addressing the origin of disorders, favouring a non-speculative standpoint. Finally, in the 1960s much sociological work drew on and developed labelling theories aligned with anti-psychiatry, critiquing the existence of mental health categorizations as normative, and professionals as agents of social control. In contrast, contemporary scholars are often (though not always) more politically moderate: mental health care is framed as protective, with many scholars criticizing the lack of access to treatment, or the existence of stigma – rather than considering the origins and (political) functions of either.

These evolutions have their limitations. Whereas data now facilitates the scrutinization of diverse categorization processes in various contexts and for different disorders, fewer substantial advances can be pointed to regarding how mental disorders *emerge* in individuals and societies, and how labelling fits into the broader social organization. A related challenge is how to capitalize on the reported improvement of methodological rigour without losing sight of the bigger picture? Dealing with the production, appropriation and social role of categories, three approaches to revitalizing the study of labelling processes can be identified in the literature. First, some studies aim to expose the socio-political arrangements in which labels are produced and diffused. Second, others strive to better understand how labels affect people, frame their troubles and define their emotions. A third strand of scholarship asks what these labels do to the societies in which they thrive – what are the broader effects of labels? We address each of these in turn in the following sections.

Socio-political arrangements and the production of categories

Who creates the words that define our mental health states, why and how? Are there socio-political configurations conducive to the creation and use of these labels? Above, we noted how the social production of categories underwent significant transformation in the second half of the twentieth century; in particular, psychiatry has lost its monopoly over such production. In the previous section we also described two approaches to medicalization, one emphasizing the influential action of powerful actors (classical medicalization studies), and the other underscoring the cultural reasons for which a human problem comes to be redefined as medical (cultural sociology of health). A slightly different way of presenting this issue is to use Eyal et al's (2010) distinction, elaborated through a study of 'autism epidemics' in different national contexts, between *'supply-side' perspectives*, according to which the development of diagnosis infrastructures causes the number of diagnosed cases to increase, and *'demand-side' perspectives*, according to which, driven by various motivations, people demand more diagnosis. We agree with Eyal et al (2010) that these perspectives should be combined, and the following points develop this further.

A first possibility lies in the inclusion of more actors in studies of medicalization, beyond psychiatry and pharmaceuticals, to gain a sense of how labels permeate a given society. Indeed, several examples exist where online patient groups (Barker, 2008), the media (Kroll-Smith, 2003), political and legal institutions (Halfman, 2019), and conservative movements (Kelly, 2014; Irvine, 1995), contribute to medicalization processes. As Scott (1990) showed with the addition of PTSD in the DSM, these arrangements can be made of converging interests between medical and non-medical groups. Scott highlighted the role of *both* psychiatrists *and* pacifist Vietnam veterans in the 1970s US, campaigning for the legitimation of PTSD, in a context when colonial wars became unpopular. Some categories, such as 'sex addiction', do not even benefit from psychiatric recognition (sex addiction was only included in the DSM between 1987 and 1994, and its 'equivalent', hypersexuality, was removed in 2013), yet remain widespread due to the converging involvements of manifold actors worldwide, from therapeutic centres to newspapers, law courts to film productions, religious movements to some fractions of the self-help industry.[7] This example epitomizes the rising power of psychology and intermediate professions (such as counsellors or sex therapists) in the social production of labels.[8] In sum, it would be reductive, today, to consider that it is only psychiatry that imposes its categories on individuals: mental health labels are produced through various arrangements – even if psychiatry retains a powerful role.

A second direction focuses on the cultural legitimacy of specific actors in the production and diffusion of labels. For example, the high prestige of medicine in Western societies, viewed as 'the steward of the "sacred" value of life' (Conrad and Schneider, 1980, p 14), allowed medicalization to develop. Looking more specifically at the growing influence of psy-discourses in Western societies, Rose (1996, p 34) elaborated the concept of 'generosity' to analyse this 'peculiar penetrative capacity' of psy-disciplines, diffusing their models of selfhood as well as practical recipes for governing the thus-constituted selves. These discourses – as with more broadly medical interpretations of certain issues – go well beyond the direct intervention of psychologists. To Eyal (2013, pp 875–876), generosity denotes how

> psychological expertise, as distinct from psychologists, is strengthened not by restricting the supply of expertise but by extending it, so that managers or educational experts, for example, borrow freely from its conceptual apparatus and draw on its methods to boost their own authority.

To summarize, in addition to the previously mentioned evolving arrangements at the core of label production, we need to inquire into the various types of legitimacy at play which facilitate some forms of label gaining traction among different social groups and institutions, recognizing these often extend beyond particular professions.

Some studies embed labelling processes in broader institutional transformations that affect the societies in which they take place. In the US, Eyal et al (2010) tie the rising number of diagnoses of autism to psychiatric deinstitutionalization. They note this has been accompanied by an expansion of the network of expertise and surveillance surrounding childhood, from a psychiatric profession focused on mental 'retardation' to a wider assemblage of professionals and parents – an institutional matrix – incorporating extended labelling options, especially as autism became a *spectrum*. This transformed not only the structure of professions mobilized around childhood but also parental expectations, further bolstered by the diffusion of autism as a popular category in Western cultures.

In Romania, Friedman (2009) studies the category 'social case' – which is used to designate patients who are too poor to be released from hospitals once recovered. This is an unofficial label, though one mobilized to justify long-term hospitalization and intensive psychiatric treatment. Friedman suggests the label can be understood as the combined result of policies encouraging deinstitutionalization (patients encouraged to leave hospitals), the impoverishment of the working class (likely to experience housing insecurity), and a vanishing welfare state leaving psychiatrists few options to help patients apart from hospitalization.

Examining institutional contexts where novel labels have *not worked* can also be instructive. Barnard (2019) offers the example of the reorganization of the French welfare administration, since 2005, through a new classification revolving around the notion of 'psychic disability'. He identifies various reasons why this reform could not be fully applied despite its legal status; in particular, the new categories did not fit pre-existing organizational routines as some people would have belonged to two or more categories, creating institutional difficulties that street-level bureaucrats could not adjust to. In all these cases, institutional nets are not only examined for their capacity to produce labels, but also to enact these in everyday life structures.

A final lead is to explore how the appropriation of labels varies from generation to generation, using a historical perspective. Maynard and Turowetz (2019) examine ethnographic depictions of diagnostic processes conducted in the US in 1972, 1985 and 2011–2015, identifying how transformations of the health sector in relation to changing conceptualizations of autism could be seen 'micro-sociologically', as patients are exposed to evolving 'narrative structures' that shape their clinical interactions. Conducting questionnaires and interviews with parents of children diagnosed with autism and psychiatrists in France, Chamak and Bonniau (2013) analyse their data depending on the age of children. In doing so, they demonstrate that from the 1990s onwards, children were diagnosed at earlier ages and parents were framed as less responsible for their children's troubles. A quantitative study by King and Bearman (2011) in California also points to changing practices of diagnosis across time. They demonstrate that children were more likely to be diagnosed if other children in their surrounding social networks were diagnosed first (the contagion effect), and that the statistical impact of community wealth on the rates of autism diagnoses changed over time. In the first stages of the 'epidemic', community wealth significantly affected diagnosis rates: wealthy people in well-endowed districts 'pioneered' the epidemic (but also modest people in wealthy districts, due to 'contagion'). Over time, however, the effect of community wealth declined, suggesting that once the label is 'out', people can access it with less inequality. Although these studies all adopt different methods to monitor historical variations and generational effects in labelling processes, each points to the ways in which the interactional practices of diagnosis intertwine with broader processes such as evolving conceptualizations of autism and local phenomena such as the 'local history' of the disorder in a given geographical area.

Thus, due to the productive effect of labels in social life, the social arrangements that fuel the production and appropriation of these labels impact the experience of mental health. This is why we need to understand (1) the broader configurations of actors through which labels emerge and circulate in societies, (2) the variable forms of legitimacy these actors benefit from, (3) the institutional contexts in which labelling processes can concretely occur and (4) the historical, and generational, dynamics at play.

The black box of performativity

How do labels fashion mental disorders and selves? How can naming emotions, behaviours or thoughts – in given social and institutional contexts – affect these emotions, behaviours and thoughts? This is the challenge raised by the performativity of language, highlighting the need to consider situations and contexts in which labels circulate. Although Foucault has had a remarkable influence on this matter, convincingly making the case that discourses and *dispositifs* contribute to make us what we are, today this exploratory line often acts as an unquestioned paradigm, especially in 'post-structural' analysis where the performativity of discourses are often taken for granted. If mental disorders embody a way in which labels, categories, diagnoses or discourses intertwine, how do these processes actually operate? We have identified four potential approaches which facilitate a closer examination of these processes. Firstly, a consideration of how categories are made use of in everyday 'mundane' interactions; secondly, how 'official' labels are drawn on and given meaning subjectively; thirdly, the notion of 'looping effects', which underline the dynamic and unstable relations between labels, their use and their 'objects'; finally, 'embodied' approaches offer a way of engaging with 'non-verbal' ways that mental health categories are constructed and experienced.

One promising approach is to inquire into the use and appropriation of mental health categories, examining how they modulate individual experiences of social life, in various spheres of social life beyond the health sector. Bröer and Besseling (2017) took this approach in the Netherlands, exploring how 'low mood' is made sense of, potentially with the label 'depression', in everyday interactions. Based on an ethnographic study of a Sicilian community in Canada, Migliore (2001) conceptualizes how notions of 'nerves' (in Sicilian, *nierbi* and *nirbusu*) are mobilized in varied manners, from justifying inappropriate behaviours to expressing moral obligations related to kin relationships. Prickett's (2021) ethnography of a Los Angeles mosque draws on Emerson's micro-politics of trouble to elaborate detailed descriptions of the iterative, nonlinear introduction of mental health-related labels within social relations. These three examples, as they look at mental health-related categories negotiated in 'mundane' situations (contexts that are not institutionally framed by health professionals), enlighten our understanding of the daily fluctuation of meanings and the social conditions in which they performatively influence the characterization of everyday issues and identities.

Another fruitful approach takes 'official' labels and their use as an object of study; dissecting the complex ways that mental health categories are taken up by groups or individuals. In their ethnography of a facility dedicated to adolescents in New Mexico, Jenkins and Csordas (2020) 'identify a field of discourse characterized by a distinct *discursive structure* and within which diagnostic terms can be understood in their function as *discursive operators*' (p 114, emphasis in original). Jenkins and Csordas propose a 'structural model' composed of four dimensions. They distinguish (1) how patients make sense of the diagnosis, which does not always align with its psychiatric meaning ('understanding'); (2) how patients develop different opinions regarding whether this diagnosis describes their condition ('agreeing'); (3) the practical utility they found in the diagnostic category to deal with their everyday life ('usefulness'); and (4) the intensity with which they use the diagnostic category in their narrative ('engagement with diagnosis'). These four dimensions are not necessarily coherent – say, someone can find their depression diagnosis very useful without agreeing that they are depressive.

A related example is Brinkmann's (2016) work which examines the social psychological processes entangled in the diagnostic process: diagnosis as an 'epistemic object' can be understood through *having* ('having ADHD' relates to an entity that someone is deemed to 'possess'), *being* ('being ADHD' relates to the identity associated with this diagnosis) and *doing* ('doing ADHD' relates to the activities associated with the diagnosis) a mental disorder. Diagnoses can then be used in an explanatory way (to give an explanation of one's issues), in a self-affirming way (to reframe one's life narrative), and for disclaiming (to claim exemption from some responsibilities). In this regard, autoethnographic descriptions, such as that of McMahon (2020) on schizoaffective disorder in Australia, are a rich resource, as they detail how labels are received, reworked and sometimes rejected – how they affect people and societies beyond a linear model of discursive influence.

One of the most epistemologically grounded concepts to deal with categorial performativity, is the notion of 'looping effects' (Hacking, 1995b) – a concept that allows consideration of how categories shape social life and experience, and conversely, how social life and experience shapes categories; looping effects are dynamic and underline the instability of labels and their meanings. This notion relies on Hacking's distinction between 'kinds', differentiating those that are not affected (indifferent kinds), completely affected (interactive kinds), and partially affected (hybrid kinds) by their social labelling; mental disorders belonging, according to him, to the last two kinds.[9] Hacking's perspective has been criticized for lacking a full conception of the self (Tekin, 2014) or of consciousness (Tsou, 2007) resulting in over-general or superficial analysis of how and under what conditions looping effects occur – similar problems have been raised about Foucault's philosophy. In sociology, this point brings us back to the methodological problem of substantiating how performativity precisely operates, or how looping effects can be observed 'on the ground', beyond attesting the social existence of a category and assuming its impact in societies and individuals. Still, the notion of looping effects remains useful in drawing attention to the dynamics at play around the labels and categories given to mental disorders.

Embodiment is another promising notion, but similarly difficult to operationalize. A slowly expanding trend within social studies of mental health relates delves into how mental health experiences – and related labels – are embodied (Bendelow, 2009). For example, Warin (2000) examined the way in which people diagnosed with schizophrenia draw on bodily experience, as well as a mixture of psychiatric and spiritual beliefs, to make sense of their condition. Engaging with bodies and embodiment, but not in a purely biomedical frame, allows engagement with culturally specific and situated ways in which bodies are understood and experienced, and therefore, how these may shape what a particular 'diagnosis' means in a given place and time. Similarly, Chandler's studies of self-injury have underlined the centrality of bodily practices in 'making up' what self-injury is and what it means. For Chandler (2016), attending to the nuanced ways in which both psychiatric accounts (in the DSM-5's attempts to delineate 'Non-Suicidal Self-Injury' as a proposed diagnosis), and individual accounts of the meaning and experience of self-injury entail taking seriously the role of bodily experiences and practices – which draw on and in turn shape (as per Hacking's looping effects) 'self-injury' as a cultural object. Many mental disorders encompass bodily dimensions, from motor slowdown in depression to inner tension in anxiety through dissociation in certain forms of schizophrenia, but they are often downplayed in sociological literature, which focuses more on words and cognitive reasonings. Thus, 'embodied' research opens up new directions in conceptualizing the performativity of mental health labels – labels without words.

To summarize, if labels, discourses, diagnoses or categories can be performative, such performativity still needs to be better theorized, and methodologically refined. All research dealing with mental health involves, in one way or another, dealing with processes of categorization, because mental health is a field structured by categories originating in psychiatry and now, in psychology. By definition, this includes implicit assumptions about the nature of these categories and their potentially performative outcomes in social reality. Authors differ in how they integrate categorizations into their theoretical and conceptual universe, evoking different visions of the self, mental health, the function of language and the power of institutions. We have sought to make this landscape of positions more explicit.

Why do labels exist?

Finally, it is time to return to an essential question: why do labels exist? What justifies, nurtures, prolongs and establishes their considerable importance in contemporary social life? Even if the word 'function' has fallen into disuse with the decline of functionalism in sociology, the 'function' of diagnosis and of labelling in societies still constitutes a major source of inquiry. Although this issue seems to have become obvious in most mental health research, it is not: after all, there is no formal necessity for humans to name, categorize and develop typologies of mental health states. Why labels exist is a constitutive ontological question, because ontologies condition how labels are understood to contribute to the social production of mental disorders.

The main debate in this area regards the necessity of diagnoses and potential alternatives to this dominant form of categorization. The worry about over- or underdiagnosis has always been present in psychiatry and social sciences (Brinkmann, 2016, pp 12–13). More substantial propositions have been suggested by Sadler (2004), Staub (2011), Pilgrim (2007) or Rose (2018): diagnoses, as inherently inaccurate reductions of human experiences, could give way to more flexible tools to help suffering people. As Rose (2018) proposes: 'from diagnosis to formulation' (pp 89–93). In 1952, Fanon talked about 'situational diagnoses'. At its most radical, the critique of diagnosis proposes the abandonment of these devices, for instance, where Mirowsky and Ross (1989), claimed that diagnoses obscure judgement rather than helping to make sense of the problems they designate. This discussion takes on different forms in the mental health sector and, in contrast to the 1960s, most professionals today are aware of the weight of labels. But here again, the debate lacks broader questions: what would non-reductive diagnoses entail in terms of care and rights? What would a world without diagnosis look like?

A striking social process, somewhat characteristic of our time, is the proliferation of labels stemming from psychiatry, psychology and other health-related professions. In parallel, diagnoses acquired an impressive range of social uses, as Rose (2018, p 73) lists, providing gateways to treatment, welfare and insurance benefits, or various professional exemptions. Although we have already addressed several approaches which account for this process, there are still broader reflections to expand upon: what does this all mean for people and societies? Recently, Busfield (2017) resurrected Ivan Illich's critique of 'medical colonization' in a review of the concept of medicalization. A priest, social theorist and activist, Illich published *Medical Nemesis* in 1974, where he attacks the whole medical institution as a form of authoritarian dominance, alienating humans by its glorification of health and technologies and through this obscuring the meaning of life. Medicine, to Illich, is no more than a facet of the capitalist apparatus in which individuals only have to be functional. People try to stay healthy at all prices to compensate the gaps left empty by capitalism, as they cannot find fulfilling purpose with labour or consumption; this applies to biomedical psychiatry and mental health. This perspective sketches a reflection on normativity and meaning at large, and this is why it matters that Illich was a priest, even a lapsed one: what is the point of using so many medical, psychological and mental health frameworks for the purpose of our existence?

In some regards, the psychiatrization of human conditions through labelling lead to individualization and depoliticization. Conrad and Schneider (1980) already made this point: medicalization processes *individualize* social problems, and in doing so, they *depoliticize* them. This was a long-lasting debate in psychiatry, as Murat (2014) explains, since revolutionaries have been deemed 'crazy' at least since the 1789 French revolution – pointing to the fine line between revolt and madness; politics and insanity. Some activities and emotions considered to be mental health problems can indeed be ambivalently interpreted as manifestations of resistance against various orders – societal, familial or political (see Brossard, 2018, pp 171–175, about self-harm). Therefore Guerin (2021, pp 76–111) suggests that instead of using diagnoses to characterize individual ailments, obscuring their contexts of production, psychologists could on the contrary use these categories to emphasize relations to contexts, and what makes these contexts potentially pathogenic. For psychiatrist Moncrieff (2010), diagnoses are 'political devices': they do not serve as starting points for designing mental health care for patients, but rather formulate an a posteriori justification of social reactions to deviance.

At an explicitly political level, today the lexicon of mental health provides a language which can serve to legitimize state governance initiatives, as Fassin and Rechtman (2009) show with Western policies based on the recognition of trauma, or Younis and Jadhav (2020) on how psychological services in the UK government's counter-terrorism initiatives tacitly perpetuate forms of institutional Islamophobia and racism. Stigma can also be instrumental, and while Goffman elaborated this concept in an apolitical manner, recent interventions from Tyler (2018, 2020), Tyler and Slater (2018) and Scambler (2018) make a strong case that stigma is 'weaponized' in the neoliberal era, meaning that it is not only a societal reaction to mental disorders due to internalized norms, but a politically orchestrated concept that naturalizes the existing economic order in blaming its victims. All in all, we should question what mental health labels do beyond the health sector, and beyond the conditions of troubled individuals: what they do to our political orders and their reproduction.

On the other side of the same coin, words can enact social transformations. At first sight, in the area of mental health, such changes tentatively occurred through the challenging of labels that carried pejorative representations (such as 'crazy' or 'retarded'), reductive descriptions of people ('people living with schizophrenia' instead of 'schizophrenics'), patronizing relationships to institutions ('patient' tends to be replaced with 'customer', 'service user' and sometimes 'survivor') or normative hierarchies ('neurotypical' *versus* 'neurodiverse'). These modifications do not always come with the transformations they strive to materialize; still, they change something. Two empirical studies provide further examples of the potential use of labels in transformative ways. Nakamura's (2013) ethnography of Bethel, a Japanese community programme built upon the acceptance of mental illness, explains that hallucinations there are referred to as *Gencho-sans* ('honourable voices', positive and accepted) and *Okyaky-sans* ('honourable visitors', out of control). Either can be collectively rewarded with the Award of the Best Hallucination of the Year. This renaming is knowingly performative, in that it changes the connotations attached to what otherwise constitutes a – strictly negative – symptom. Note that the efficacy of such an initiative does not come from labels alone, it relies on institutional routines (such as the award), and contextual conditions such as, according to Nakamura, progressive mental health policies, individual initiatives (such as psychiatrists willing to get involved in this atypical project), Christian traditions (evoking a culture of charity) and an economy in crisis lowering real estate prices, which in concrete terms allowed the Bethel community to acquire some buildings. Another example is Snedker's (2016) study of US mental health courts. Using Collins' interaction ritual theory, Snedker advances that the setting of the court creates the conditions for emotional energy to arise and destigmatize the accused through its ceremonial features: the court, with all its folklore, makes a ritual arrangement that give strength to the transformative use of mental health categories.

Conclusion

Labels do not solely qualify mental health disorders. They contribute to producing these disorders, generating the material and symbolic worlds that people – diagnosed or not – inhabit.

Woman at the Edge of Time, Piercy's novel which we drew on at the start of the chapter, offers powerful and insightful examples that illuminate the implications of naming things: labels structure reality, and they can carry conservative forces as well as utopian visions. Discourses, categories, diagnoses are not good or bad in themselves but for the space of possibilities they open. As such, especially at a time when much research shows that psychiatric and psychological classifications rely less on some unshakeable 'science' than on various contingencies, the political undertones of labelling should become a crucial area for future reflections: what do the categories available in a given society tell us about this society? What would labelling processes look like in institutions driven by social justice? In the political system we wish to experience – say, democracy – how should we ideally and practically characterize differences and vulnerabilities?

This conclusion leads us to question the sociology of mental health as a field *specialized in* the study of the mental health apparatus. Such specialization runs the risk of missing significant issues, no less than the part effectively played by categorizations in social life at large. The sociology of mental health, in fact, should be thought of as a form of political sociology: who labels whom, how, with what power, in what institution, and with what legitimacy? How do these labels fragment societies into classes, groups and scales? The dynamics through which some people are designated, what legitimizes these designations, and the influence of these processes over social structures indeed falls within the scope of politics both in its broadest and strictest sense. In other words, how labelling processes occur and 'make up' mental disorders inherently relates to how societies deal with their divides, their order and, eventually, their transformative waves.

4

The Uses of Culture

> In my childhood I often happened to see and hear these 'possessed' women in the villages and monasteries. They used to be brought to mass; they would squeal and bark like a dog so that they were heard all over the church. But when the sacrament was carried in and they were led up to it, at once the 'possession' ceased, and the sick women were always soothed for a time. I was greatly impressed and amazed at this as a child; but then I heard from country neighbours and from my town teachers that the whole illness was simulated to avoid work, and that it could always be cured by suitable severity; various anecdotes were told to confirm this. But later on I learnt with astonishment from medical specialists that there is no pretence about it, that it is a terrible illness to which women are subject, specially prevalent among us in Russia, and that it is due to the hard lot of the peasant women. It is a disease, I was told, arising from exhausting toil too soon after hard, abnormal and unassisted labour in childbirth, and from the hopeless misery, from beatings, and so on, which some women were not able to endure like others. (Dostoevsky, 1998 [1879], p 94)

In his novel *Brothers Karamazov* (1998 [1879]), Dostoevsky makes a detour with this portrayal, combining several themes that occur when one addresses the entanglement between culture and mental disorder. Disputed meanings of 'madness' are at stake here, present in three coexisting interpretations of women's distress. Some say the 'possessed' women suffer from a medical condition, a disease to be treated by doctors. Others speculate that these really are in fact cases of possession, and the women should be cared for by the *starets*. Or perhaps instead they simulate such affliction to avoid work. Dostoevsky anchors his description to a particular sociocultural context: exhausting peasant work, childbirth in difficult conditions, and additional hardships, misery and beatings, supposedly typical of Russia, which might generate this *singular* state of being. Although similar troubles exist elsewhere, what is 'cultural' here is left to interpretation.

A multitude of research projects have led to the conclusion that a deep connection exists between 'culture' – this panel of shared meanings, symbolic worlds and material environments in which individuals of the same group are socialized – and 'mental health' experiences (Luhrmann and Marrow, 2016; Kirmayer et al, 2017). In medicine, some initiatives appeared to explore this connection, such as 'transcultural psychiatry', made possible 'when colonial conditions afforded doctors the possibility of observing mental illnesses in colonized peoples according to western psychiatric concepts' (Delille and Crozier, 2018, p 257).

Studies of mental illness and culture have had some striking results. Some troubles, such as *amok*, *nervios* or *ghost sickness*, exist only in some places and not in others. Other disorders, at first glance, look similar anywhere on earth, but may manifest themselves through different symptoms. When people in the US hear voices, they are more likely to be confronted with violent and intrusive words than Indian and Ghanaian people, who develop more diverse relationships with their inner speakers (Luhrman et al, 2015). A textbook case is depression: intense sadness in the West is said to be experienced much less physically than in China, where bodily symptoms are a more important part of how depression is identified and experienced (Kleinman, 1977).

The recurrent observation that mental disorders are not the same from one geographical and cultural area to another has been used to suggest that disorders are rooted, to a large extent, in the sociocultural conditions in which they emerge. Put another way, if the causes of mental illness were purely biological, and uninfluenced by sociocultural context, we would expect their prevalence rates and symptoms to be the same everywhere, which is not the case.

For more than a century, anthropologists and cultural psychiatrists have dug into the challenges carried by this observation (Littlewood, 2001). They asked whether aspiring to understand the problems of the 'others' inherently amounts to reducing these others to their cultural alterity, or whether any analysis unavoidably bears the seal of the culture of the one who performs the (mis)interpretation. In the history of sociology, consideration of culture has been quite irregular, but always present under the form of generalizations about 'Western', 'modern', 'developed', 'neoliberal' or 'post-industrial' societies: the society of the one who writes. Often omitted are the exclusive implications of these words, drawing a vague fissure, setting aside whole civilisations. Underlying these questions lie the problems of dealing with alterity, universalism and cultural relativism in social research.

In the early twenty-first century, the mental health literature seems torn between three *uses of culture*. Firstly, there are approaches which conflate culture with race, ethnicity or religion to characterize the experiences, practices and accounts of migrants or minority ethnic groups in the Global North, drawing on 'culture' as an explanation for mental distress and disparities. Second, culture can be used as a way of characterizing a Zeitgeist, especially in the 'West': culture here is used loosely to refer to, for instance, 'culture of consumerism' (Bauman, 2007), or, more controversially 'a culture of poverty'. A third, divergent use of culture instead focuses awareness of the colonial dynamics that structure the production of knowledge in general (Visweswaran, 2010), and psychiatric biomedicine in particular (Hernández-Wolfe, 2011; Mills, 2014; Horn, 2020; Fernández and Gutierrez, 2020). In this context, it became necessary to take stock more broadly of what we know about the cultural origins of mental disorders and – crucially – how we (think we) know this.

This chapter first introduces pioneering works that established connections between psychiatric disorders and culture, before presenting the main current theoretical positions on this matter, structured around the inclusion of 'culture-bound syndromes' in the DSM-IV. Then, we identify ways in which social scientists associate culture and mental health in contemporary research: in showing how mental disorders reflect certain cultural trends (the 'diffusion', 'inversion' and 'amplification' reasonings) or in seeing individual relations to their culture as a potential factor in the development of mental disorders (the 'clash', 'consonance' and 'loss' reasonings). Towards the end of the chapter, we turn to critical propositions on how social scientists can renew their engagement with the notion of culture. On the one hand, inspired by anti-psychiatry, neurodiversity, mad studies and disability studies, we sketch emerging avenues that approach mental health beyond the 'deficit narrative'. On the other hand, we critically examine what we call 'integrative models', such as bio-psycho-social models, decolonial theories and Hacking's theory of ecological niches; these models, despite their inherent methodological problems, might constructively reinvigorate the notion of culture as a jumpstart to complexify the social studies of mental disorders.

Cultural explanations: birth of a research question

In a field where 'madness' has frequently been conceptualized as representing 'prior' evolutionary and civilizational stages, the reassessment of our academic legacies through the lens of colonialism becomes both urgent and inescapable. Since the colonization of the Americas, Africa, Asia and Oceania by European powers, many psychiatrists (Cohn, 1996) and anthropologists (Stocking, 1991) have been involved, intellectually and practically, directly or indirectly, in the facilitation of colonial governance. This ranged from being directly involved in ruling colonized peoples (Linstrum, 2016), to discrediting independence movements by psychologizing them (Pringle, 2019, pp 93–116; Pols, 2018; Cohen, 2014, pp 187–192). This history can be excavated from and identified in cultural conceptualizations of mental health that have surfaced over time, for instance, via attempts to differentiate 'Western' and 'non-Western' selves (Kusserow, 1999), elaborating a 'colonial subject' (Anderson et al, 2011), little by little installing racialized structures of knowledge production (Bhambra and Holmwood, 2021).[1]

It is quite ironic, however, that such reassessment often takes the shape of an enlightenment narrative whereby some colonial past is progressively replaced by a state of greater awareness, separating a before and its villains, such as ethno-psychiatrists (McCulloch, 1995), and today's heroes – 'us'. This narrative fails to recognize broader and nonlinear initiatives to make sense of alterity that compose the history of anthropology (Weber, 2015). Nor does it hedge against the resurgence, in postcolonial thinking, of essentialism, or 'new culturalism' (Visweswaran, 2010). Thus, we will outline some seminal steps in the elaboration of a cultural approach to the psyche, underscoring the complexity of works which de facto result from colonial conditions of knowledge production, while their authors adopted much more critical positions towards this context.

A socialist and committed critic of capitalist colonialism (Mallard, 2018), Marcel Mauss played a significant role in the development of social sciences. In the 1920s, he attempted to convince psychologists to abandon their medical view of the mind and instead consider what he called the 'total man', that is, the human taken as a whole, in its biological, psychological, and social dimensions (Chevance et al, 2021; see also Mauss, 1979; Ignatow, 2012). He did not convince them. Still, his contemporaneous writings had major implications for the social understanding of 'psychology'. In 'The obligatory expression of feelings', Mauss (1921) demonstrated that feelings are not natural reactions to social settings, but that culture demands its members experience and express emotions in a certain manner. In 'The physical effect on the individual of the idea of death suggested by the collectivity' (Mauss, 1926), also based on reports from colonial Australia and New Zealand, he shows that the transgression of certain social expectations can lead physically healthy individuals to die out of mere self-suggestion. In addition to setting the scene for the sociology and anthropology of emotions, these arguments paved the way to later conceptualizations of the performativity of rituals (see Levi-Strauss, 1949) and critiques of the mind/body divide on which cultural approaches of mental health are now founded (Williams and Bendelow, 1998).

Meanwhile, on the other side of the Atlantic, following the footsteps of Franz Boas – an early theorist of cultural relativism – the 'culture and personality' school gathered anthropologists and psychoanalysts around the study of how personality and psyche are constructed in relation to the cultural environment in which they arise (Bains, 2005). A key figure of this movement, Ruth Benedict (1934a) defined culture as the patterned behaviours and ideas to be found in a group, as well as the socialization mechanisms by which they stabilize. Her cultural relativism was both humanist and pragmatic. While Nazism spread in Europe, promoting racial hierarchies, she claimed that activities found in different cultures share a concern with common human problems,[2] an idea that unfolds in her critique of (the omission of) colonial dynamics in social sciences:

> The psychological consequences of this spread of white culture have been out of all proportion to the materialistic. This world-wide cultural diffusion has protected us as man had never been protected before from having to take seriously the civilizations of other peoples; it has given to our culture a massive universality that we have long ceased to account for historically, and which we read off rather as necessary and inevitable. (Benedict, 1934a, p 6)

Although the findings of the 'culture and personality' school were limited, and strongly criticized for their reductionism (one culture = one personality), they did provide a basis on which later research could elaborate links between culture, personality and mental disorders. The works of Margaret Mead (1928), for example, became emblematic of the possible cultural variations in socialization and their effects on phenomena previously deemed biological, such as puberty and sexuality.

Around the Second World War, especially in its aftermath, two notable trends appeared in scholarship on cultural explanations of mental disorders: one that integrated the role of colonization in individual psyches and social suffering (Balandier and Fanon), the other that proposed social psychological theories of mental illness with a concept of culture at their core (Devereux and Bateson).

Although to our knowledge, Georges Balandier never directly wrote about psychiatric disorders, he considered colonial societies as pathological in themselves, which deserves a few words. Conducting fieldwork in Sub-Saharan Africa, Balandier refused to be the anthropologist of ever-lasting traditional cultures, and rather claimed to be a *sociologist* of 'the colonial situation' (Balandier, 1951). His portrayals of colonized societies depict social change through European intervention as disruptive, painful, not solely because African peoples could not live up to their traditions, but because they were dispossessed from their own social, economic and political fate (Balandier, 1970).

Frantz Fanon conceptualized the effect of colonization on mental health more explicitly. A psychiatrist, activist and writer from Martinique, Fanon's critique of psychiatry was twofold. The first, laid out in *Black Skin, White Masks* (1952), accuses psychiatry of relying on a universalized vision of the human mind that is, in fact, that of white European elites. Thus the Oedipus complex, a pivotal notion in the then-dominant psychoanalytical framework, would only work for individuals being in a social position of dominance. For the Oedipus complex to develop, Fanon argues, children shall be able to represent themselves through their own ideals, not those fixed by others. In this specific context only can individuals have their own family as a space of unconscious fantasizing. This is not the case for colonized subjects who grow up with the images of the others, the colonizer, as material and symbolic references. Their fantasizing horizon is elsewhere. Therefore the Oedipus complex, so to speak, is the privilege of the dominant. It does not apply to black and colonized peoples, like most psychoanalytical concepts. Fanon's second critique is clearly formulated in 'North African Syndrome' (1967), in which Fanon attacks the French psychiatric system where 'the North African, spontaneously, by the very fact of appearing on the scene, enters into a pre-existing framework' (Fanon, 1967, p 7). Importantly, this critique cannot be reduced to the mere unveiling of situational discriminations, to be resolved with a handful of well-intentioned policies: it questions the very construction of the psychiatric apparatus as a colonial device.

Let us turn to the other trend previously announced: explanatory models of mental illness based on culture. Born in current Romania, Georges Devereux, an ethnologist and therapist, foreshadowed ethno-psychiatry, theorizing the intertwining of psychoanalysis and anthropology through cultural factors, with his main essays, written from the 1930s to the 1960s, gathered in *Basic Problems in Ethnopsychiatry* (Devereux, 1980). Devereux attempted to integrate indigenous knowledges in Western psychoanalysis, for instance in respect to the aetiological role of dreams. His posterity remains associated with the controversial idea that shamans are the 'equivalent' of Western psychotics, sharing symptoms but differing in the social roles they have been attributed by their group (Luhrmann, 2000; Stephen and Suryani, 2000); though in contrast his 'sociological theory of schizophrenia' was forgotten. This theory characterizes schizophrenia as a form of disorientation that arises in 'complex' cultures where knowledge is excessively specialized. Those with schizophrenia are individuals who try to grasp this overwhelming complexity by making generalizations based on narrowly selected empirical facts. Schizophrenia, less than a disorder of the persons, would then be a side effect of 'modernity' (Devereux, 1939).

Gregory Bateson formulated a different theory of schizophrenia in the 1950s: the 'double bind' theory. According to Bateson, schizophrenia emerges when someone finds themselves in a relational system composed of repeated contacts where one regular injunction contradicts with another one, more abstract, and this person cannot escape such configuration. Later Scheper-Hughes (1977) used this theory in her study of 1970s rural Ireland, where sons of farming families were expected both to stay home and take care of their estate and also 'succeed', which involved, in a context of dire economic crisis, emigration – an impossible situation. As for Devereux, schizophrenia in Bateson's (1972) work connects with the complexity of modern life.

From the beginning of the twentieth century to the post-war era, many working hypotheses circulated about the relation between culture and mental health (summarized by Leighton and Hughes, 1961). In these earlier studies, culture is said to shape mental disorders by: producing basic personality types, some of which are vulnerable to disorders (Benedict); in encouraging socialization that would shape later mental health problems (Mead); legitimizing social control that formalizes norms, transgressions and frustrations (Fanon); rewarding pathological prestigious statuses (Devereux); generating stressful situations and roles (Bateson); generating emotions that can later make the material of mental disorders (Mauss) or disturbing individuals with social change (Balandier). These hypotheses were later nuanced, while psychiatry adopted a more reductive approach to culture.

Culture-bound syndromes, Western biomedicine and relativism

In the decades following the Second World War, several social processes transformed the ways in which mental health and culture relate to one another.

Western psychiatry has unfurled its worldwide influence. Authoritative categorizations such as the DSM and ICD, which aimed to reference all diseases to be found anywhere around the globe, sought a legitimacy that expanded beyond the limits of the former colonial empires. The elaboration of several psychotropic drugs opened a market into which pharmaceutical industries stepped, now a fully-fledged part of the psychiatric enterprise (Moncrieff, 2007; Whitaker, 2011; Giraldi, 2017). Relatedly, 'scientific' approaches took precedence over psychoanalysis, except in a few countries such as France or Argentina. The spread of independence movements sparked awareness, in social sciences and beyond, of the colonial dynamics at play in the health sector (Lewis, 1973; Cooper, 2004). Psychology and intermediate disciplines, such as counselling or sexology, prospered in relative independence from psychiatry. Taken together, 'psy-discourses' turned into a form of soft power in globalized, neoliberal economies (Rose, 1996), where cultural variations often became mere anecdotal curiosities that would mask the real, core pathologies that affect humanity at large. 'Global mental health' emerged as a political project, actively promoted by some international institutions such as the World Health Organization, and diffusing three – debatable – arguments: (1) high rates of mental disorders can be found in all cultures; (2) this 'reality' is 'hidden' by insufficient diagnostic structures in many countries; and (3) the solution is to 'scale up' mental health services from the West to 'help' these countries (Summerfield, 2012, 2013; see also Myers, 2010; Mills, 2014).

It is not an exaggeration to say that during this era, mainstream psychiatry and psychology often delved into blind triumphalism, asserting their universal, scientific understanding of mental health issues (while these issues dramatically soared 'on their watch'). In contrast, social sciences quietly added cultural experiences, globalization contexts and the complexity of causes into the study-kit of mental health scholars (Jenkins and Barrett, 2003). However, disagreements exist regarding the *extent* to which mental health is 'cultural' and three approaches stabilized towards the second half of the twentieth century.

The universalist position argues that mental disorders constitute universal realities which apply to anyone, wherever they live, wherever they were socialized, wherever they come from. Mental disorders correspond to dysfunctions of the brain or troubles in mental life that humans thus share beyond borders, and to which culture-related manifestations give various shapes – but without changing their core nature. In this perspective, culture is only a varnish.

This position, stereotypical of biomedicine, and which peaked in the 1990s (Luhrmann and Marrow, 2016, p 2), tends to be suggested rather than asserted. Many publications indeed start from the latent premises that mental disorders are universal, as they do not differentiate these disorders depending on the contexts in which they thrive. Some adopt more explicit, global health assumptions, for instance stating that 'depression is the leading cause of disability worldwide, yet in many cultures, it remains unaddressed and unacknowledged' (Williams et al, 2018, p 194). Others advance that Euro-American institutional devices should be implemented in non-Western contexts, on the grounds that their measured efficacy could be replicated anywhere with minor 'cultural' adjustments, framing cultural specificities as potential difficulties to be ironed out (Ferrazzi and Krupa, 2016). Similar questions regard the use of standardized psychological scales, whose translation into different languages engages very technical debates on cultural linguistics, but not on the possibility that the meaning of mental health could fluctuate, beyond words, from one region to another (Matías-Carrelo et al, 2003).

Driven into a corner by the findings of cross-cultural psychiatrists and anthropologists, the universalist position is sometimes refined in the light of clinical experience that most symptoms look alike anywhere in the world (Patel and Winston, 1994). Still, this position has become difficult to support in view of the accumulating observations that fundamental differences separate what constitutes 'madness' in various contexts, and that some of these clinically documented similarities themselves result from the deliberate initiative of Western organizations (Watters, 2010; Mills, 2014).

Kleinman offers a 'reversed' anecdote to explain why one should beware the raw observation of symptoms in different contexts:

> Suppose some psychiatrist in South Asia, where semen loss syndromes are common, traveled to the United States, where these syndromes have neither professional nor popular coherence. Let us imagine that this South Asian psychiatrist has first operationalized the symptoms of semen loss in a psychiatric diagnostic schedule, translated this interview protocol in English, had other bilingual persons translate it back into the original language to check the accuracy of the translation, adjusted those items that were mistranslated, and then trained a group of American psychiatrists in its use and established a derive prevalence data for 'semen loss syndrome' in the United States. But would these findings have any validity in a society in which there are neither folk nor professional categories of semen loss and in which semen loss is not reported as a disturbing symptom? ... regrettably, much of cross-cultural psychiatry has been conducted in a rather similar manner (but by Western psychiatrists). (Kleinman, 1991, p 15 drawing on Obeyesekere, 1985)

The *split-relativist position* contends that while some mental disorders remain universal as their incidences appear equivalent around the globe,[3] others are specific to cultures, such as *susto* or *latah*, or their symptoms change so dramatically that 'culturally-tailored' interventions are needed, such as for depression and anorexia. The American Psychiatric Association (APA) endorsed this position, in including 'culture-bound syndromes' in the DSM-IV (APA, 1994). This posture also increasingly permeates global mental health organizations, which call for the consideration of local idioms of distress and the respect of local traditions (Mills, 2014; Kidron and Kirmayer, 2019).

Another feature of the split-relativist position consists of the visualization of mental disorders, metaphorically speaking, as universal epicentres around which some cultural layers would filter the expression. Let us take the example of depression in Iran. According to Behrouzan (2015), the normalization of the term *dépréshen*, ﺪﭘرسﮔی ﺎﻓسﺮدﮔی, should be seen as a tension between the psychiatrization of human distress typical of Western psychiatry and the memories of the Iran–Iraq war, especially among the generation who was young during this war, in the 1980s. On the same topic, Mirdamadi (2019) advances that a specific 'death-consciousness' structures a singular way of experiencing depression in Iran, also heavily affected by the war with Iraq. Both works stress how the reality captured by a Western category 'depression' is *coloured* by historical and cultural experiences, while the fundamental aspects of its nature withstands.

At first sight, the acknowledgement of culture-bound syndromes in the DSM looks like a U-turn from the universalist framework that characterized previous classifications. However Arthur Kleinman (1997), one of the most prominent figures of twentieth century US anthropology of mental health, warned against this 'Pyrrhic victory': culture-bound syndromes are relegated to a glossary housed in Appendix 9, strictly separated from the main body of the DSM-IV where the epidemiology and expression of disorders remain 'culture blind', which ultimately reinforces the divide between the universal/Western and the cultural/others. In addition, measurement methods did not change but for peripheral elements, for which arguments become circular: how do we measure cultural variation using diagnosis tools generated in a particular cultural ('Western') milieu? In this perspective, ethnocentrism is only reconfigured, made more diffuse.

The *radical relativist position* posits that the very notion of 'mental disorders' cannot be exported outside the West because it is the local production of Western psychiatry. Lutz (2004) offers a good illustration of this approach. Comparing 'Euro-American culture' and that of the Ifaluk, a people living in the Federal States of Micronesia, she demonstrates that both cultures differ not only in their definition of depression, or what could be its 'equivalent' for Ifaluks, *fago*, but in their conception of emotions. While Westerners may feel sadness for itself, with no particular reason, Ifaluks experience *fago* in a relational way: they are sad of something, because someone did something to them, in the frame of a link to someone, through love or out of compassion; these two words, love and compassion, can also translate *fago*. Ifaluks cannot be sad as Westerners are. Thus, can they suffer from depression if their emotional repertoire does not integrate any equivalent of sadness? And what about 'mental disorders', the definitions of which dissociate emotions from their relational origins, completely out of phase with the Ifaluk relational approach to feelings? Diagnosing depression among the Ifaluks would therefore fall within ethnocentrism: it mobilizes a representation of emotions and diseases relevant only to the Global North. By the same token, most Westerners would find it unsuitable to be diagnosed with *fago*.

Whereas the relativist position seems to best integrate the state of knowledge in contemporary anthropology, the worldwide diffusion of psychiatry and psychology might challenge its longevity. Summerfield (2012) provides various examples of this process, such as how the organization Multicultural Mental Health Australia developed a campaign targeting Afghan refugees to help them 'learn' about depression and antidepressants, using the Fari word *mualagh* to reach this audience. At length, even symptoms potentially uniformize. Watters (2010) shows that whereas anorexia in China included distinct symptoms in the 1990s – Chinese anorectic young women were not disgusted by food as Westerners were – Chinese psychiatrists started to report forms of anorexia similar to the West in the 2000s. Under this movement, mental disorders might become universal indeed.

People within cultures: diffusion, inversion and amplification

In the eighteenth century, a new disorder sailed into France. A far-away ancestor of depression, the Spleen was imported from across the English Channel. Prominent intellectuals, no less than Voltaire, would write about their travel to England and their curious realization that, there, the Eastern winds put populations under the threat of a violent form of melancholia. Such importation was bolstered by the prestige of England, then a pioneer on the political and economic scene, and migration movements, often fleeing away from religious discrimination, who carried with them the representations of their country of origin (Hansen, 2009). In one century, the Spleen became a French disease. Not only did people declare the same symptoms as their British counterparts, but it turned into a local cliché with the publication of Baudelaire's poems collection, *The Spleen of Paris*, in 1869.

This example begs several questions. How do mental disorders 'circulate' from one culture to another? Does this circulation flow with existing balances of powers? What is the temporality of such circulation – for instance, why do diagnoses persist in some places, yet fall out of favour in others? (See Pinto, 2014 on hysteria in India.) Then, in which elements of culture do 'new' mental disorders take root? In contemporary literature, these questions mostly concern the Westernization process and how mental disorders are embedded in and produced by this process. These reflections can be summarized in three ideal-typical reasonings: (a) 'dominant' cultures *diffuse* idioms of distress; (b) mental disorders reflect the *amplification* of the values, attitudes and representations promoted in a given culture; and (c) disorders consist of the *inversion* of values, attitudes and representations found in a culture.

The diffusion model considers that a culture deemed dominant exercises such an influence that it can also 'export' its mental disorders.

In the 1990s and 2000s, eating disorders became the prototypical illustration of this process, as these disorders, initially identified in Western contexts, started to be discovered all around the globe. A 2004 special issue of *Culture, Medicine, and Psychiatry* crystallized the resulting debates. To Lester (2004; see also 2007) and Littlewood (2004), that anorexia and bulimia can be observed in Mexico exemplifies the diffusion of post-industrial neoliberalism. Important refinements were also proposed. Pike and Borovoy (2004) agreed that anorexia expresses a state of global capitalism, but noticed specific adaptations in Japan, in view of singular gender roles and beauty standards. In Curaçao, a Caribbean country, Katzman et al (2004) reported that women who suffer from anorexia share notable common points. They aspire to be part of the mostly white, mobile elite, distancing themselves from the black majority, having the means to stay overseas and get the education to envision this form of mobility. Therefore, both advance that cultural influence, or Westernization, does not occur uniformly but involves local adjustments and affects some groups more than others.

Whereas Western psychiatry is associated, worldwide, with a form of 'modernity', the examples of Lebanon (Abi-Rached, 2020), China (Baum, 2017), Argentina (Bonnin, 2020) and Uganda (Pringle, 2019) show that local therapeutic techniques and idioms of distress variably persist yet in distorted forms. Ng's (2020) study of Chinese psychiatry adds that such 'mixes' fluctuate with political eras: some traditional healers affirm that ghosts and demonic spirits disappeared during the reign of Mao, 'a hiatus for spectral stirrings' (p 126), but resurfaced after his death (when Western psychiatry started to progressively permeate China). Thus, interestingly close to the critiques of diffusionism already present in Benedict's (1934a) writings, some scholars now moderate the Westernization model. At a time when countries such as China, India or Brazil take a growing role in the 'concert of nations', these nonlinear processes of adjustment might be worth exploring more.

In the amplification model, people with mental disorders are analysed as paroxysmal figures, pushing some traits of their culture to an extreme.

Emily Martin's (2007) *Bipolar Expeditions* contains elements of this reasoning. While stigmatized as a form of madness, bipolar disorder also triggers admiration for the creative potential it unleashes. Martin examines how the media portrays successful entrepreneurs and artists as people whose success partly draws on their 'manic' energy. The social imaginary of a delicate balance between success and risk of forfeiture – including suicide – carries the ideal of the entrepreneurial individual in a perpetually manic state; such emotional instability echoes contemporary changes in work management, promoting flexibility, adaptability and creativity. The case of autism, and its fantasized association with 'genius' (Murray, 2008), or that of 'gambling addiction', a 'paradigmatic form of consumption that captures the intensified logic at the heart of late modern capitalist societies' (Reith, 2013, p 717), offer other illustrations of this model.

The inversion model contends that symptoms of mental illness are the reversed image of cultural norms that dominate a given society. For instance, Ehrenberg (1998) draws parallels between characteristics of Western societies and depressive symptoms. He argues the 'epidemic' of depression emanates from novel configurations of social and cultural life in the twentieth centuries, when 'modern' life is no longer governed by tradition. Rather, individuals are expected to build their own identity, 'becoming themselves', but the ransom of liberty is high: 'identity insecurity'. Depression, according to Ehrenberg, here close to Giddens (1991), reflects a failure to fulfil these sociocultural ideals, as it embodies the 'weariness' of those who cannot live by these standards.

Moreau (2009) furthers this perspective and analyses depression in relation to temporality, drawing on interviews with people who define themselves as 'depressed' and/or who take antidepressants in Canada. With changes in capitalist organizations and modes of management, a majority of individuals passed from having their time structured by others (as per Taylorism) to the injunction to self-organize (via flexible schedules in start-up companies) – from 'external' to 'internalized' social control. Through their symptoms, people suffering from depression embody, both mentally and physically, the opposite of these rising cultural norms. Instead of leading their lives at a fast pace, choosing their own succession of tasks, they are demotivated, physically tired, and do not display a strong sense of their achievements; medicines as tools of social normalization put them 'back on track'.[4]

A similar but more straightforward reasoning is developed in Han's (2015) analysis of burnouts as a result of the changing modes of production. Here again, mental illness represents an inversion of dominant cultural norms: they are the illnesses of those who 'fail' to follow.

All these models rest on the possibility of associating 'elements' of a culture with the symptomatology and representations surrounding particular mental disorders: but how are these associations constructed? Some of the above-mentioned authors investigate *discursive resemblances*, or what, in the discourses produced in a culture – for instance in the media, resonates with the symptomatology of the disorders under study (see Martin, 2007, and the image of the bipolar entrepreneur). Others prioritize *structural resemblances*, namely what, in the economic or political transformations to be identified in a given society, mirrors the symptomatology of a given disorder (such as Moreau, 2009, and the temporality of work and depression). That certain disorders affect *certain groups more than others*, or in different ways, can also tell us about their relation to culture(s) (Katzman et al, 2004, on the social profile of women suffering from anorexia in Curaçao). Finally, these models concern *conditions of possibility*:[5] finding in the specificities of a culture some elements *without which* a disorder would not be possible.

Counter-factual argumentation has been used straightforwardly by Littlewood and Dein (2013), who assert that Christianity was a condition of possibility of schizophrenia. It can also be found in Steggals (2015), who argues for neoliberalism as a condition of possibility for the forms of self-harm practised by young women in late twentieth/early twenty-first century Britain; and Greenfeld (2013), who suggests that the main mental disorders diagnosed today, schizophrenia and depression, are the by-products of the rise of egalitarianism since the sixteenth century.

Cultures within people: clash, consonance and loss

Another way in which 'culture' is understood to produce mental illness raises attention to individuals' relations with the cultures they are exposed to throughout their life. Three models of reasoning can be found: clash, consonance and loss.

The 'culture clash' model implicates the struggles of migrant groups when adjusting to the culture of their new country of residence in producing distress.[6] The difficulties of migration and identity-related matters – the 'double absence', as Sayad (2004) put it – are well-known, even among second and third generations. Today, many works examine the health outcomes of migration, or having 'foreign origins'. For example, Gulbas and Zayas (2015), arguing for an 'experience-near' examination of cultural – through familial – influences on mental disorder, follow the identification of high rates of self-harm among Latin American young women in the US. Carrying out interviews with Latina teens and their parents, they contrasted accounts of families where Latina teenagers had experienced self-harm or suicidal behaviour, and where they had not. The crucial difference related to emotional isolation: in families where suicidal behaviour was not an issue, teens did not report emotional isolation in the same way. Gulbas and Zayas argue:

> Latina teen attempters are 'betwixt and between assigned cultural positions' ... Without the tools to bridge her transcultural worlds, the young Latina feels isolated and alone ... With nothing left to help her deal with her suffering, she might succumb to behaviors aimed at self-destruction. (Gulbas and Zayas, 2015, p 696)

Gulbas and Zayas attribute the emotional isolation to particular challenges faced by *Latina* teens in navigating a 'cultural contradiction'. However, research with young people from a range of cultural backgrounds who have experienced self-harm and suicidal behaviour has identified family tensions and emotional isolation as well (Chandler, 2016; Brossard, 2018; Steggals et al, 2020). How can emotional isolation per se be attributed to a lack of fit between 'transcultural worlds'? How does a focus on this feature explain the disproportionately higher rates of suicidal behaviours identified among young Latinas? Wider structural conditions arguably shaped such isolation and the very fact that 'cultural contradiction' was formulated by participants as a problematic experience in the first place: migratism, racism, sexism and so forth (Collins and Bilge, 2016; Tudor, 2017). Thus the 'culture clash' model runs the risk of psychologizing historical and political constructs of culture, and develops a view monolithic on this concept, implying that humans need unilateral affiliation in order to experience wellbeing.

The *cultural consonance model* was formulated at the turn of the 2000s around Dressler (et al, 1998). 'Cultural consonance is the degree to which individuals, in their own beliefs and behaviors, approximate widely shared cultural models' (Dressler et al, 2007, p 195). To investigate this concept, Dressler and colleagues seek qualitative features of culture understood to be significant (attitudes towards food, towards social support, and number of material good owned) and turn these features into questionnaire items and quantified indicators to examine correlations between self-reported distress, or signs of disorder, and the extent to which individuals endorsed these cultural ideals. A key finding from Dressler et al's (2007, 2016) studies is that the more 'consonant' people are with the standards of their culture, the less likely they feel psychological distress, and by extension suffer from mental health issues. This association has been measured and corroborated in various contexts, from Amazonia (Reyes-García et al, 2010) to New England (Maltseva, 2018).[7]

Culture(s) place(s) people in contradictions, which makes the clash and consonance hypothesis converge. This is, for example, the approach held by Shorer et al (2018), exploring the subjective experience of PTSD among indigenous Bedouin veterans of the Israeli army.

> This cycle [of isolation and trauma], in which culture serves as a 'double-edged' sword, encompasses two key contradictory aspects in the life of the injured Bedouin veteran: belonging to a traditional collectivistic society and being a wounded Israeli soldier. (p 773)

A similar conclusion is developed by Dengah et al (2019) about women in Utah, both religious – Mormons – and secular, as they suggest that conformity to one model provides mental health benefits whereas trying to fit with several increases stress.

While the previous position remains close to the traditional sociology of deviance, in which deviance (including mental disorders) entails some discrepancy with cultural norms, some works point to the other direction, towards the *excess* of consonance as a driver of mental distress, evocative of Durkheim's altruistic and fatalistic suicides. Developing this perspective, Mueller and Abrutyn's (2016) work in a small affluent community in the US characterized by high rates of youth suicide concludes that intense social networks might generate excessive expectations, in the sense that individuals might always feel as acting 'under the eyes' of the community, thus embodying overwhelming pressures to perform – with suicide a culturally recognizable response to such pressure – see further theorizations in Abrutyn and Mueller (2016, 2018). One could therefore extend the consonance/clash reasoning to two kinds, one marked by several cultures with contradictions that alienate individuals, and one where, in contrast, too much integration in one culture makes its expectations distressing.

Finally, *the cultural loss model* applies to peoples living in a situation of dramatic change, mostly due to Westernization and colonization. Mental distress is then provoked by the loss of bearings, attachment and symbolic benchmarks. Wexler (2006) advances that suicide among the young Inupiat of Northwest Alaska – one of the highest rates in the world – can be understood through the historical oppression that led to the progressive loss of the Inupiaq culture and society. Self-destructive trends are formulated as an outcome of the disintegration of community. This model can also be applied to Western societies that, far from being at the brink of extinction, still lost many of their traditional organizations and community customs under the weight of capitalist economy,[8] and the ecological crisis might further change the situation (Cunsolo and Ellis, 2018).

The cultural 'clash', 'consonance' or 'loss' models have the merit of not conceiving culture as an essential, static individual feature, as they represent people more or less successfully fitting into one or more evolving cultures. However, some recurrent limitations remain: the methodological difficulty of delineating and operationalizing cultures in quantity and/or in quality; the difficulty of accounting for variable meanings of mental distress proper to each culture; and a persisting tendency to view those moving 'to' a place as 'other', and the culture of the place they move to (often the US) as the neutral 'normal', or the *non-cultural*. An ultimate issue is that these approaches rely on the quite conservative idea that a mentally healthy person is one who has no cultural conflict, comfortably sitting in one's culture, where people moderately incorporate the same values and attitudes.

Contemporary perspectives on 'culture'

The concept of culture addresses the overall meanings and symbols to which people are socialized in relation to their material conditions of life. Its strength is its weakness. On the one hand, it offers a fertile, encompassing perspective on the social environment in which individuals come to suffer from mental illnesses and in which mental illnesses develop as collective phenomena. On the other hand, the adjective 'cultural' can also become, as Lester (2004, p 609) puts it, 'something of a catchall term for anything not strictly psychological or biological,[9] and as a way of displacing concerns that might otherwise require a more profound examination of the cultural bases of the diagnostic criteria themselves'. In view of the issues observed in the literature, we will sketch three essential points to consider before turning to future-oriented propositions.

First, *everybody has 'culture'*. If culture broadly refers to systems of shared meaning and practices, in association with elements of social structure such as stratification and the organization of kinship, then everybody has culture. This statement sounds flatly obvious. However, as Luhrmann (2007) also notes, many publications use this term when describing the singularities of 'other' people, reintroducing in silence a Great Divide in our journals and our minds. Typically, while Westerners are deemed to have opinions, lifestyles and representations, non-Westerners tend to be depicted as abiding by 'cultural values', such as in Afghanistan (Eggerman and Panter-Brick, 2010), Nepal (Kohrt and Bourey, 2016) or Taiwan (Tzeng and Lipson, 2004; Lee and Kawachi, 2017). The same applies to migrants and racialized groups (Visweswaran, 2010). Caution should be exercised, too, when 'cultural' relates to the difficulties health professionals face when working in multicultural settings (Granek et al, 2020), who would then need 'cultural competence' (Olcoń and Gulbas, 2018). In public health, there is a fine line between developing an understanding sensitivity to alterity and convincing foreign or indigenous populations of the merits of one's standpoint. Despite the long history we summarized in this chapter, the use of 'culture' does not go without saying, and Brown et al's (2013) call to better articulate race, ethnicity, nativity and cultural influences in mental health research provides a potential solution to the problem.

Second, *cultures are composite epistemological entities*. Another major issue indeed lies in the 'monolithic' conceptualization of culture that prevails in many mental health studies. As Takeuchi (2016, p 430) puts it, 'culture in health studies tends to be operationalized as static and uniform for a particular group', for example, as a set of clear-cut worldviews and attitudes. However, cultures are configurations of potentially conflicting institutions and meanings: cultural dimensions exist only within a field of contradictions. The omission of this point can lead to misleading generalizations. For example, Picone (2012) shows that the 'cultural dimensions' of suicide in Japan, often attached to the image of the honour suicide – the famous Harakiri – originate in attitudes found only in the old warrior class, that is, 6 per cent of the Japanese population, exclusively men. Acknowledging that culture is realized through concrete institutions, such as family, school, religion or work, or that 'social institutions are the primary anchor of the fit between culture, structure, and psyche' (Jacobs and Spillman, 2005, p 4, citing Derne), may offer a way out of excessive generalization. Also, sociological research engaging with 'subcultures' has generated telling studies of certain communities, in majority young people, who adopt appearance and consumption patterns in affiliation with a range of overlapping subcultures. Some interesting lines of flight focused on 'goth' subcultures, associated with higher rates of self-harm (Young et al, 2006) and 'metal' subcultures, where membership was said to protect against distress (Rowe and Guerin, 2018). In short, several methods point to uses of the notion of culture without dismissing the complexity of environments in which people live.

Third, *cultures are, more than discourses, discourses embedded in geopolitical dynamics*. This means that any representation, narrative, worldview or mindset identified as cultural cannot be fully understood without reference to the geopolitical processes in which it emerged. Especially, this caution applies to the 'post-structural' interpretation of Foucault's work, which rightly highlights that discourses shape selves, but where do these discourses come from, and what concrete power relations make such shaping possible? Graeber (2004) criticized Foucault for paying too much attention to discourses in themselves, forgetting how money, institutions, weapons, diplomatic relations and quests for prestige are often involved in the imposition of words. Discourses cannot be considered without the material structures of their enunciation. Research operating at the global scale enlightens this point; for instance, the promotion of the trauma paradigm and talking therapies by Western NGOs in Sri Lanka after the 2004 tsunami, which ignored local cultural beliefs that recommended not talking after a catastrophe to prevent spirits invasion, was enabled by significant material means and cultural prestige (Watters, 2010). Asking *whose* concepts researchers and participants use ('trauma', 'recovery' or 'cultural values') to think about mental health, as well as *where* these concepts and worldviews come from, *how* they were adopted, *when* and *under what circumstances*, and where 'culture' sits in all this, is a good start.

Illness as cultural expression

> It is perhaps ironic that we learnt our most profound lesson about consciousness in rural South Africa from a madman ... Famous for an ingenious costume that he would never remove, the man was, literally, a prophet in polythene robes. His crazy clothes spoke the language of his obsession. His boots, standard issue for mineworkers, were topped by intricately knitted leggings, the painstaking product of many unraveled orange sacks. He wore a cloak and a bishop's mitre, fashioned from black plastic garbage bags. Across his chest was stretched a brilliantly striped sash, on which were stitched three letters: SAR. For his white attendants, these were the most obvious signs of his delusion, although they noted that he also 'heard' things. The other patients, however, regarded him as an inspired healer, sent to them in their affliction. SAR was his church, and he its sole embodiment. The letters stood for South African Railways, alongside whose track the hospital lay. In fact, at the very moment we encountered him, the night train for Johannesburg rattled by with its daily cargo of migrants. Later, as we puzzled to decipher his message, we kept returning, as he did, to SAR. It was a message that spoke directly to his fellow inmates and also to the black paramedical staff. For, in this world of peasant-proletarians, the railway forged a tangible link between rural and urban life, hitching together the dissonant worlds of the country and the city. (Comaroff and Comaroff, 1987, p 191)

At first sight, this excerpt from the Comaroffs' (1987) ethnographic work in South Africa is reminiscent of the amplification model: through the display of various symbols, the 'madman' embodies his changing culture to its extreme. But another articulation of mental illness and culture can be extracted from this portrayal. As the Comaroffs hint, such staging *teaches a lesson* 'about consciousness in rural South Africa'. It is an entry into the history of this country, if not an eroded expression of lucidity.

Several research trends have shifted away from the 'deficit narrative' – seeing mental illness only as a problem – to an epistemological status of meaningfulness. In the 1960s and 1970s, the anti-psychiatric movement reimagined the social role of madness and its experience in a positive light, such as an inner voyage (Crossley, 1998) or an emancipatory vanguard mindset (Cooper, 1971, 1978). This approach has been accused of romanticizing both mental illness and its difficulties (Luhrmann, 2000), especially as it taps into the common sense association between mental illness, creativity and genius (Becker, 1978; Kaufman, 2014; Kyaga, 2015). More recently, mad studies and disability studies built upon a similar but less whimsical critique of the deficit narrative, advocating the integration of disabled people, or those living with mental illness, into research and policy and contesting the psychiatric monopoly over the understanding of mental illness (Ingram, 2016; Gorman and LeFrançois, 2017).[10] In the same vein, even if often deploying a binary divide between the neurodiverse and the neurotypical, the proponents of 'neurodiversity' carved the image of a pluralist society that citizens would inhabit with, or even through, their neurological differences (Rose, 2020; McWade et al, 2015; Kapp et al, 2013; Ortega, 2009).

These sources of questioning prompt us to elaborate on the approaches that consider mental diversity and 'madness' beyond problems that should be cared for by welfare systems and therapeutic devices, and beyond the weaknesses they occasion or are attached to. As we will see, symptoms can be taken as forms of expression through: 1) the atypical appropriation of cultural objects; 2) the processing of traumatic history; 3) the collective problematization of mental life; 4) the realization of an expressive potential; or 5) the manifestation of an ethical stance towards the world.

Much like the Comarroffs' (1987) portrayal, mental illness can be read as the singular staging of 'cultural objects', in resonance with specific aspects of political and social history. Leuenberger (2006) gives the example of how German psychology used the Berlin Wall as 'interpretive resource' and 'narrative object' to analyse the psychology of German people. In each historical generation of therapists and patients, the German Wall evoked different memories and were integrated differently in existing symptomatology, from constituting a fully-fledged pathology, the 'wall disorder', to the 'wall in the head' metaphorically designating psychological disparities between the two Germanies after 1989. Investigating admissions in nineteenth century French mental hospitals, Murat (2014) notes that a significant number of psychiatric patients believed that they were illustrious figures, and especially Napoleon Bonaparte. Asking why people would fantasize about being Napoleon rather than others – say, Louis XV or Robespierre – Murat speculates that common traits bound psychosis and Napoleon's personality, notably his usurping attitude and quite delusional *folie des grandeurs*. In Turkey, Rahimi (2015) theorized schizophrenia as a form of distorted use of culturally situated networks of association that mirror Turkish history, such as Atatürk's reforms (which initiated the Westernization and secularization of the Republic of Turkey). Napoleon, Atatürk, the Berlin Wall: in all cases, mental illnesses appear as the products of an unexpected way to symbolize these 'cultural objects'; reminiscent of Deleuze and Guattari's famous approach according to which, 'when unraveling into delirium, the unconscious does not play around with mommy and daddy, but with races, tribes, and continents, history and geography, always within a social field' (Deleuze, 2013, p 162; our translation).

A nascent trend in cultural sociology revolves around the concept of 'cultural trauma'. Cultural trauma occurs when a social group collectively experiences an adverse situation, rephrased in a narrative, which structures the very identity of this group. Alexander et al (2004) developed this notion and applied it to various populations, from Holocaust perpetrators to African Americans, with the trauma of slavery (on the latter case, see Eyerman, 2001). Without necessarily employing the concept of cultural trauma, several works approach mental health issues as generational challenges constitutive of identities, especially for war veterans (see Fitzpatrick, 2017 about Korean war trauma in North America) and following catastrophes such as 9/11 (Neria, Gross and Marshall, 2006). Thus certain cultures would be prone to psychological difficulties (Scheper-Hughes (1977) called 1970s rural Ireland a 'broken culture'), a point taken further with the rise of epigenetics, which has had strong resonances among the First Nations of Australia (Warin et al, 2020). In these cases, mental health issues stand at the foundation of generations and groups, if not 'nations'; they express the collective processing of the aftershock of history.

Let us turn to mental illnesses as related to thinking processes. From 'lack of hindsight' in schizophrenia to fragmented focus in ADHD, from obsessive rehashing in PTSD to suicidal ideation in depression, through the multiform pathologization of 'thinking too much' in several regions of the world (Kaiser et al, 2015), mental disorders represent instances of mental functioning deemed abnormal, unhealthy or troublesome. They are a collective problematization of mental life, situated in 'the psyche'. Additionally, from meditation to psychotropic drugs, from anxiety management applications to behavioural therapy, most techniques supposed to increase wellbeing imply a direct action on their users' stream of thoughts. Surprisingly, although the theoretical foundations of North American sociology rely on a conceptualization of the mind as a social process, empirical explorations of this dimension of social life are lacking (Ruiz-Junco and Brossard, 2018; Schweingruber and Wahl, 2019). There is the need for more work, especially with the rise of the neurodiversity paradigm, on the variable understandings of the mind (Luhrmann, 2020), of 'cognitive deviances' (Zerubavel, 1997), or the 'autonomization of thoughts' (Brossard, 2014) and their sociocultural production in relation to mental health.[11]

The idea that symptoms of mental illness might help maintain the stability of a relational configuration, once elaborated upon by the Gestalt and Palo Alto schools of psychology, has been taken over in some sociological research (but without the notion of stability). Billaud (2012) emphasizes the 'communicative potential' of Afghan women's suicide, that both conveys 'cultural ideas' about femininity and its inner weakness, and simultaneously challenges the masculine honour system in voicing discontent. Billaud qualifies and situates female suicide as 'a covert form of protest, a performance'. Similarly, Steggals et al (2020) highlight the communicative dimension of self-harm in the UK, characterizing this as an ambiguous, 'absent presence' – contrasting with narratives about self-harm which emphasize secrecy and silence. Like Chandler (2016, 2018), these works point to the complex, culturally and socially contingent – sometimes contradictory – ways in which mental health experiences may be both 'performed' and made sense of. In this frame, mental health issues 'propose' a different way to relate to the others, expressing some messages that cannot be formulated otherwise, inexpressible but socially meaningful: they say what a culture makes unutterable.

Finally, what if mental disorders express an ethical stance? The environmental crisis has led many social scientists to reconsider the anthropocentric epistemology at the basis of their disciplines. In mental health, this resulted in the design of categories dedicated to the characterization of suffering attached to the Anthropocene, from 'ecological grief' (Cunsolo and Ellis, 2018) to 'solastagia' (Albrecht, 2005). These considerations might go in the direction of Guerin's suggestion to privilege 'direct social action instead of individual therapy' (Guerin, 2021, p 43). These emerging approaches reshape mental distress as not resulting from individual weakness but from adverse conditions that involve more than trauma or stress: a quite understandable form of empathy, or an ethical relation to the world.

Towards integrative models

A key challenge we encounter in the study of culture and mental illness is a tendency towards over-simplification, neglecting intricacies and the porous boundaries that always blur what we put in the word 'culture'. Uses of culture are inherently criticizable as they bring together facets of reality that do not neatly combine in a slick construct. Nonetheless, insightful and convincing causal links connect culture and mental health, as we have shown. For these reasons, integrative models – models that incorporate multiple dimensions of social life and mental health – may point to productive paths. We will discuss three reasonings: 1) bio-psycho-social models that aim at integrating elements of biological into social perspectives; 2) Hacking's theory of ecological niches, which formulates a way of simultaneously considering several elements of social context often studied separately; and 3) post- or decolonial perspectives that advocate the inclusion of colonial dynamics as a way of rethinking social studies of the coloniality of mental illness.

Bio-psycho-social models

The integration of biological features has triggered long debates in social sciences, from Mauss' (1921) ambition to study the 'total man' to Scheff's (1966) critique of the bio-psycho-social representation of the human. In the twenty-first century, rare but increasing attempts to examine the articulation between genetics, biology, neurosciences and social sciences have furthered this pursuit (Pickersgill et al, 2013).

Theoretical initiatives include Horwitz's (2007, 2016) redefinition of the normal and the pathological, which aimed to reconcile sociology and psychiatry through the superposing of two axes, cultural and biological; for instance, incest would be both biologically dysfunctional and culturally sanctioned, while cowardice would be biologically natural and culturally discouraged. However, this analysis still depends on the social criteria that qualify biological dysfunctionality; for instance, it is because reproduction was long seen as the (social) basis of biological functionality that homosexuality was deemed unnatural.

Seligman and Kirmayer (2008) reflect on dissociative experiences. They suggest bridging the 'psychiatric-adaptive' paradigm, where dissociation is a reaction to trauma, with the 'anthropological-discursive' one, where dissociation occurs through socially sanctioned rituals, let alone the fluctuations of daily consciousness that sometimes involve transient forms of dissociation. They argue that 'the patterns of neural activation that produce the experience of dissociation are a result of a complex interaction among proximate causes, like trauma, and more complex sociocultural and cognitive processes' (Seligman and Kirmayer, 2008, p 51).

Advancing a 'cortisol sociology', Roberts and McWade (2021) propose 'critical triangulation' to refine the inter-relation between the biological and the social through meanings, and the emotional and bodily realties at play. In all cases, the problem remains interpretation: how to interpret neural activation, biomarkers or biological substances – taken alone, these indicators cannot inform about any emotion or pattern.

Another difficulty concerns the empirical exploration of these possibilities. Biological and physical anthropologists elaborated several studies in this area. McDade (2002) measured antibodies against the Epstein-Barr virus as a biomarker of psychosocial stress among Samoan people and found that the level of these antibodies was higher in cities than in rural areas. He concludes that in this historical context where Western influence primarily impacts urban areas, Westernization provokes stress. Another example is provided by Dressler et al (2016), who, armed with questionnaires and swabs, studied the interaction between some genes associated with depression (polymorphism in the 2A serotonin receptor), childhood adversity, cultural consonance in family life (or cohesion within family) and socioeconomic status, in an urban community in Brazil. They conclude that some genes made people more vulnerable to childhood adversity, the outcome being depressive symptoms in adult life, and that this correlation becomes stronger in lower socioeconomic classes. But this correlation almost disappears in families with greater cultural consonance.

In these examples, it is striking that such sophisticated measurements reproduce common sense assumptions: life is more stressful in big, Westernized cities than in the traditional countryside, and childhood adversity is better managed in cohesive families with sufficient economic means. And, again, the interpretation of biomarkers remains subject to what researchers construct as worth measuring.

Ecological niches

Hacking's theory of ecological niches opens an interesting way of combining several elements of social context. With his notion of 'looping effects', Hacking (1995b) developed a useful tool to understand how categorizations and mental disorders as realities intertwine. Further, he proposes a theory that would explain the emergence of 'transient mental illnesses', namely, 'a mental illness that appears at a time, in a place, and later fades away' (1998, p 1; Brossard, 2019 argues to extend it to all mental disorders). Based on his epistemological stance, dynamic nominalism, to understand the 'very possibility of transient mental illnesses' (Hacking, 1998, p 1), Hacking uses the metaphor of the *ecological niche* to designate a social configuration composed of four converging 'vectors' that set the possibility for mental illnesses to emerge and flourish:

1. *Medical taxonomy*: the set of behaviours and emotions attributed to the illness should be integrated within the medical conceptions of the period, such as psychiatric classifications.

2. *Observability*: the disorder should be visible and interpreted as a problem. Logically, no mental illness could socially exist without being observable by at least some fraction of society.
3. *Cultural polarity*: 'the illness should be situated between two elements of contemporary culture, one romantic and virtuous, the other vicious and tending to crime' (Hacking, 1998, p 2).
4. *Release*: 'the illness, despite the pain it produces, should also provide some release that is not available elsewhere in the culture in which it thrives' (Hacking, 1998, p 2).

Hacking's privileged cases are the epidemics of dissociative fugue that broke out in Europe in the late nineteenth century (1998) and multiple personalities in the 1980s USA (1995a): for each he showed how these 'epidemics' corresponded to troubles that could be included in medical classifications (vector 1), observed due to specific social devices, such as border control for fugue (vector 2), refer to already-existing stereotypes without fitting with any of these (vector 3) and express some unique escape from the conditions of life of the sufferers (vector 4). To be sure, many works try to provide a comprehensive overview of the sociocultural context in which a disorder emerges, but this particular theory helps to organize this quest.

This model presents mental illness as a latent possibility activated when some social processes converge to provide its conditions of existence. It is integrative in the sense that it enables the combination of several, potentially contradictory, aspects of a culture and articulates these into a causal interpretation of mental illness. It has been applied more or less strictly to several cases, such as porn addiction (Taylor, 2019), and elaborated upon either theoretically (Murphy, 2001; Tekin, 2014) or sociologically to include the micro-social dimension of niches: Moreno Pestaña (2006) develops the concept of 'threshold' to account for how individuals 'enter' each vector and eventually fall sick; Brossard (2019) attaches this theory to several methodological and theoretical traditions in sociology. It is worth noting that the four main ways of explaining the emergence of mental disorders in sociology presented in this book are included in this model, which considers individuals' social position, how labels of mental illness appear and are applied to people, how stress and emotions operate, as well as elements of culture.

Postcolonial and decolonial approaches

How can sociologists rethink mental health through colonial dynamics, in particular (re)evaluating some elements of indigenous worldviews, dismissed if not erased by biomedical psychiatry and psychology? In the footsteps of Fanon, postcolonial and decolonial approaches provide another integrative model because they see cultures as fields of conflict, in which researchers act by their relation to knowledge; and address human psyche as a site of political struggle where traces of histories intersect (Ansloos and Peltier, 2021). Beyond denouncing indigenous stigma and colonial politics, they call for the distinction between colonialism, or the political process of colonization, and coloniality, which designates more broadly the cultural logics emerging out of colonialism, structuring our social worlds and laying the conditions for contemporary capitalism to thrive.

In current decolonial literature,[12] there are two ongoing lines of exploration. The first documents colonization and decolonization as political processes shaping local mental health care systems and the cultural references that frame the understanding of emotions and troubles. Turner and Luna Sánchez (2020) show how Mayan communities in Guatemala struggle with postcolonial politics, intertwining Northern and local notions of individuality and wellbeing. Pringle (2019), retracing the history of psychiatry in Uganda, explains how Ugandan psychiatrists both conserved elements of Western psychiatry while 'Africanising' their approach. Horn (2020) narrates the work of a feminist organization intervening in a Congo hospital to contest Western, depoliticized understandings of mental health; particularly, she highlights how PTSD individualizes the effects of violence on women, which prevents the therapeutic process being transformed into an initiative that could reintroduce the core issue of power to understanding trauma, and the agency of women in provoking social change.

The second direction deconstructs Western psychology and psychiatry, either in showing how they remain tied to colonial references and assumptions (see Coe, 2021, about Australian policy) or in reintroducing indigenous philosophies as valid knowledge to be taken into account. Dudgeon and Walker (2015) list the conceptions of wellbeing they identified among indigenous Australians, conceptions that prioritize connections to 'nature' and to community, and invite psychologists to question their own assumptions about psychology and mental health in this light. Sepúlveda Jara and Oyarce Pisani (2020) adopt a similar reasoning with the Mapuche of Chile, for whom *itrofill mongen* refers to 'human being within a chain of living beings that interact deeply with the rest of nature and the sprits that exist in them' while *Kimelkalen*, close to *itrofill mongen*, is 'based on egalitarian social relations and reciprocity' (p 336). Inspired by some Amerindian people's philosophy – but also Guattari – Souza Prado (2020) summarizes that an 'ecosophical' praxis of care, which especially contests the separation of humans from their environment, would be a condition to realize the decolonial project.

Increasingly popular, the decolonial project is only starting. In that, it still needs some clarification. Firstly, given that many states in the world expanded *manu militari* or through 'soft power' at some stage of their history, what makes a people 'colonized'? This question is not so simple: are people in Brittany (France), Northern Ireland (UK), Tibet (China), Catalonia (Spain) or Siberia (Russia), or Roma (Europe) or Tuaregs (Saharan states) colonized, and by whom? Then, who is not colonized, since any state apparatus, in a sense, reduces the culture of its people(s) to common words and rules? Also, how can we approach colonization beyond the European-centric assimilation of white people with worldwide power, especially in view of other administrations who relied on colonial expansion in recent history, such as the Chinese, Russian, Israeli, Japanese, Ottoman, Saudi Arabian or Ethiopian states? Finally, in suggesting that each 'people' should live by its own traditional rules, do decolonial theories necessarily essentialize the boundaries of national and even tribal groups, as per the nineteenth century, nationalist ideal that each people could become one with the administration of their ancestral territory?

Despite these issues, decolonial scholars fundamentally call on us to address, in the chains of causality that link mental health to culture, the effect of state-sponsored expansionist policies not only as a 'political context', but a pervasive, cultural force that fashions the most innocent facets of our concepts, and the most intimate aspects of our mental life.

Conclusion

Were these women really sick? Let us return to Dostoevsky's excerpt presented in the introduction. We omitted an important point: the place of the narrator. Dostoevsky's narrator is 'told' about the situation of the possessed women. He is 'impressed' with this information. 'But later on *I learnt with astonishment from* medical specialists that ... it is a terrible illness' (Dostoevsky, 1998 [1879], p 94, emphasis added). By this literary technique, Dostoevsky disengages the speaker from his own text. To what extent does the narrator believe in what he hears and says? Is his intention to tell the reader about nineteenth century rural Russia, its folk beliefs or its actual afflictions? Or does he rather express some ironic distance on his own 'astonishment' in the face of conflicting gossips? While the relation between culture and mental health was clearly productive in the history of social sciences, the ambivalence of Dostoevsky's narrator echoes the difficult position in which social scientists still find themselves in this regard: the difficulty of acknowledging both the multitude of material conditions conductive to mental health issues, such as farming in the hostile plains of Russia, and the meanings arising from these conditions, such as the discordant beliefs and hearsays that frame the social existence of mental disorders.

To be sure, labour in nineteenth century Russian plains was tedious. But is that difficulty specific to Russian culture, its cold weather and singular mode of production? Or are all adverse working conditions comparable, so that Bolivian workers would experience the same kind of suffering? These questions illustrate that underneath the debates surrounding the notion of culture always stands the moral and philosophical problems of universalism and alterity – while the earlier question runs the risk of essentializing Russian culture, the latter might dismiss its uniqueness. This is the dilemma also raised by decolonial scholars and, to some extent, the proponents of neurodiversity: how to consider, at the same time, that humans are equal in principle, while acknowledging their difference, without reducing them to these differences nor reifying these differences? (And in our case, differences of culture combine with differences of mental health states.) The solution is not as simple as granting more recognition and political power to disadvantaged groups, whether colonized or neurodiverse – which would still be a first step. This dilemma points to the difficulty of imagining what non-segregational differences would look like, and establishing a 'cosmopolitan' framework in which conceptualizing culture and mental health inequalities would not necessarily have the reductionist and potentially stigmatizing connotations they may evoke in our present context of knowledge production.

Conclusion: Explaining the 'Mental Health Crisis'

Every four years, the US National Intelligence Council (NIC), known for its ties to the Central Intelligence Agency, releases a report outlining the main changes to be expected in the world in the next two decades. Following this tradition, after the election of Joe Biden, a new report was published in March 2021: *Global Trends 2040*. It includes a short mention of mental health.

> Mental health and substance abuse disorders increased 13 percent during the past decade, principally because of increases in population and life expectancy but also because of the disproportionate prevalence of mental illness among adolescents. Currently, between 10 and 20 percent of children and adolescents globally suffer from mental health disorders, and suicide is the third leading cause of death among people between 15 and 19 years old. Health experts project that the economic cost of mental illness worldwide could exceed $16 trillion during the next 20 years, with much of the economic burden resulting from lost income and productivity as a result of chronic disability and premature death. Preliminary research suggests that because of the pandemic, people in every region will experience increased rates of mental distress caused by economic losses and social isolation stress disorder. (NIC, 2021, p 23)

Three causes are evoked for the rising prevalence of mental disorders: population growth, probably because it induces an increase of the absolute number of people living with mental illness, adolescent suffering and COVID-19. Most, if not all policy documents we could find approach mental health as a growing, costly problem for which few responses exist except recruiting more specialized professionals, making mental health services more 'effective' and 'accessible', and, tacitly, responsibilizing populations to manage their own distress – with increased focus on building 'resilience' and promoting 'recovery' (Harper and Speed, 2014). 'Evidence-based' policies then evaluate the 'efficiency' of these programmes and keep the most cost-effective ones, ignoring that beyond the help and relief these services certainly offer for many people suffering from mental disorders and their relatives, at a societal level, diagnosed mental disorders keep rising everywhere, no matter how cost-effective such services are.[1] Other 'factors' are at play.

This book has provided insights into the wealth of research that explores the multiple social roots underlying those experiences that manifest as mental health issues. Such a vast array of research contrasts dramatically with the intellectual poverty found in policy documents. Social sciences do not often come up with 'turnkey', institutional fixes – this being the work of policymakers. However, they produce multiple leads to understand the broader mental health situation and its social conditions of production and possibility, which necessarily move beyond the problem-solution dichotomy. This is because the theories and methods of the social sciences suggest that *mental health is not about mental health*. What appears as a mental disorder, or mental distress, is the visible façade of much deeper social processes. As such, any solutions we might offer may not square with the established frameworks of 'mental health' policies at all.

Following these observations, two solutions appear. Either the NIC asks us to rewrite the report, which seems unlikely, or we explore how the reorganization of research outlined in the present book could draw alternative understandings of the *'mental health crisis'*; showing how the considerable expertise accumulated throughout decades of research in social sciences contributes more fully to explaining mental illnesses; and – therefore – how this could inform responses to the current 'crisis'.

Social trends

'Mental health crisis' is an expression commonly used to describe the high, and increasing, prevalence rates of most mental disorders, either in particular countries or in the world. This rise acquires dramatic proportions as, if the current trends continue, the *majority* of people living in Western countries will be diagnosed with at least one mental disorder in the course of their life. In this regard, the COVID-19 pandemic was an accelerator more than an event. In the UK the volume of calls received by mental health services exploded during the first months of the pandemic (Campbell, 2021) as prevalence rates of many disorders, depression in particular, rose from the already high 10 per cent to 20 per cent (Williams et al, 2021). Let us briefly review some evocative figures for the UK, US and Australia.

In the UK, the Mental Health Foundation gathers statistics from varied academic sources to portray the mental health situation of the British population.[2] It is estimated that about one adult in six suffers from a mental disorder. Depression, anxiety, schizophrenia and bipolar disorder are the main diagnoses reported, in order of importance. Almost 20 per cent of the population reports experiencing symptoms of anxiety or depression.

The estimated lifetime prevalence[3] of depression in England is 4–10 per cent. The one-week prevalence of generalized anxiety in England is 6.6 per cent. There are almost 4 million cases of mood disorders (including bipolar disorder) in the UK, which makes 6 per cent of the population. Suicides approximate 6,500 per year (8 per 100,000).

In Australia, the Blackdog Institute (2020) monitors mental health research and, combining related statistics, suggests that 20 per cent of Australians aged 16–85 report experiencing mental illness. The most common issues are anxiety disorders (14 per cent), depressive disorders (6 per cent) and substance use disorders (5 per cent); they overlap, which explains why the total of these percentages make more than 20. Additionally, 6 per cent of the population is estimated to have bipolar disorder. Suicide is the leading cause of death for Australians aged 25–44 and second cause of death for young people aged 15–24 – around 3,000 deaths a year, with a rate of 12.5 per 100,000.

In the US, the National Institute of Mental Health states that 'mental illnesses are common in the United States. Nearly one in five US adults live with a mental illness (51.5 million in 2019)',[4] with a 49.5 per cent lifetime prevalence for young people aged 13–18 years. At some point of their lives, 7.1 per cent of all US adults have experienced a major depressive episode. Lifetime prevalence is 8.7 per cent for ADHD, 2.2 per cent for anxiety disorder and 6.8 per cent for post-traumatic stress disorder (PTSD). Suicide is the second cause of death among young people aged 10–34 years, and its rate is 16.1 per 100,000 in general population.

In high-income countries, in general, people kill themselves more often than they kill others. In the US, there are two and a half times more deaths by suicide than by homicide. In most of the Global North, the discrepancy is even higher. What does this mean?

These numbers, though debatable in many respects, illustrate well what the mental health crisis indicates: that serious amounts of people claim to experience behavioural troubles and emotional distress, and that an impressive web of institutions and services – what we sometimes call the 'mental health apparatus' – is deployed to monitor, define and respond to their suffering. The size of the crisis is measured by the concerned governments, if only for the sake of economic planning. Thus, in Europe, it is estimated that mental health issues 'cost' economies between 2 and 5 per cent of their annual GDP, including an average of 1.3 per cent spent in mental health services (OECD, 2018, pp 19–43). In the world in 2020, 80 per cent of national health insurances now include reimbursement schemes for people with mental health conditions (WHO, 2020, p 57). These numbers express large-scale realities, let alone individual sufferings.

These individual sufferings have a collective shape. If they were purely individual, then their rates would be completely random, oscillating as individual dramas come and go. If these singular distresses were not related to one another, the percentages previously mentioned would shift from one year to another, like a roller coaster. However, the trends sketched above present striking regularities. Both rates and types of disorders follow mostly continuous curves, consistently rising, crossing national territories. Everywhere in the West, depression and anxiety are the main reported mental health problems, more women are diagnosed with the latter, and if, of course, some discrepancies remain, such as in the autism 'epidemics' for which some US states have significant differences (Eyal et al, 2010), it is still within an overall 'epidemic'. How might we explain this global phenomenon that, as the NIC suggests, would cost US$16 trillion worldwide in the next 20 years?

In the following sections we draw on the four themes of this book in order to generate a sociologically informed understanding of the 'crisis'.

Pathogenic dominations

For almost a century, research conducted on mental illness and social position has confirmed, unsurprisingly, that inequalities are detrimental to mental health, in the sense that poverty and deprivation leads to a higher probability of developing emotional and behavioural problems. Similarly, that the higher people are situated in the social hierarchy, the more protected they are from mental distress is a well-known correlation. This means that mental health is intimately entangled with modes of economic production, social divides and inequalities. Increases in the prevalence of most mental disorders can thus be partly interpreted as an effect of rising inequalities (Wilkinson and Pickett, 2009; Piketty, 2017), especially structural inequalities and adversities associated with economic crises and austerity policies (Mills, 2018): the more poor people in a population, the more people suffering from mental illness, as deprivation leaves people more vulnerable. For instance, in the UK, we mentioned that the prevalence of depression increased from 10 per cent to 20 per cent during the COVID-19 pandemic, but this figure reaches 37 per cent for the poorest fractions of the population (Williams et al, 2021).

A mental health crisis is a crisis of inequalities. There is a considerable amount of evidence for this proposition. This implies that mental health policies miss a significant part of the problem they strive to address by detaching their area of action from the economic policies that produce inequalities, as well as from the set of institutions, such as school systems or corporate management, that give these inequalities their ubiquitous cultural meaning and material impact. We delineated three ways of going further.

From an *intersectional perspective*, inequalities are materialized and experienced differently depending on how they combine to make singular identities and attendant relationships with power (Collins and Bilge, 2016). Here again a strong trend appears quite clearly in the literature: members of dominated groups suffer from more mental health issues than the rest of the population, and disadvantages generally worsen one another. In other words, women, LGBT+ people, members of racialized groups and those living with a disability report higher rates of mental distress, with some exceptions raised in Chapter 1. Thus, in addition to economic hardship, broader social divides have an effect on mental health through social identities – belonging to a disadvantaged group or claiming a minority identity comes with its share of pressure. How can we interpret this observation in view of the mental health crisis? If mental health partly results from the array of social factors that intersect in the making of social identities, then the mental health crisis as a social phenomenon partly reflects the landscape of identities in which individuals are (problematically) positioned. It echoes a world of differences, tolerance, competitiveness and stereotypes. It has something to do with how culture provides us with frames to make sense of our position in the social world, and to seek recognition for the identity associated with this position. While contemporary Western countries are far from being the most discriminatory, they are shaken by intense debates, if not struggles, around the cultural recognition, legal acknowledgement and historical roots of these identities. From this standpoint, the mental health crisis could be read as manifesting a general concern with identity and social position, in which some 'intersections' ultimately lead people to be more affected by the power dynamics and oppression taking place in their society and, by extension, more vulnerable to mental illness.

The *configurational perspective* designates an approach to social position where people are inscribed in a network composed of various groups and statuses. It highlights that individuals are rarely immersed in one uniform milieu; they instead inhabit composite situations where individuals holding several positions interact. One way to read the mental health crisis in light of the configurational perspective is to posit that people who experience inequalities, differences and stereotypes through daily interaction in these configurations might live with an uneasy sense of their place in society. For example, they might find themselves in situations where they face contradictory injunctions due to their acquaintance with several social spheres, or where their position appears problematic, as Brossard's (2018) study of self-injury exemplifies. Even taking a more quantitative perspective, Lee and Kawachi (2017 T) found symptoms of depression were correlated with socializing with people who are wealthier. They proposed that exposure to the injustice or unfairness of wealth inequality was a potential driver of this correlation; at the very least suggesting that inequalities affect people differently depending on the social configurations in which they socialize. This provides a potential mechanism for Wilkinson and Pickett's (2009) arguments about the role of inequality *in general* driving poor health (including mental health) across all strata of society.

Although the studies we grouped under the term 'configurational perspective' provide more of a methodological approach than a macro-social theory, one can also speculate that the mental health crisis might correspond to the multiplication of certain composite configurations that place people within multiplying – competing or jarring – expectations, which would entrench potentially 'pathogenic', socially produced relational patterns (see also Freund, 2010).

The *definitional perspective* implies that the very definition of mental disorders targets some groups, or publics, contributing to the reproduction of certain aspects of social stratification. Typically, women are deemed more depressed, men more autistic: the ghosts of feminine melancholy and male genius hover around our heads. Therefore, mental disorders can be understood as a medium through which sets of norms attached to some positions, or differences, are legitimatized, naturalized. From this perspective, the mental health crisis can be seen as a result of the rising match between multiplying and changing psychiatric categories with their equivalent in terms of social position. This is what Cohen (2016) advances with the US American Psychiatric Association's Diagnostic and Statistical Manual (DSM), strengthening, version after version, its gendered and productivist expectations through lists of symptoms. Does this imply the tightening of social norms defining the contour of each social identity, such as being a woman or a man, a worker – especially for those who cannot work – a student or a family member? In this regard the mental health apparatus plays a multifaceted role: sometimes it reinforces capitalist and traditional injunctions over people; sometimes it also accompanies social transformations, supporting changing gender expectations and 'work–life balance', as both recently became areas of concern in psychology. In any way the mental health crisis has something to do, again, with the expectations surrounding social positions, their potential stabilization and narrowing, and productivity in neoliberal economies and cultures. Perhaps it is no coincidence that we see a tightening of gendered and productivist expectations at a time where gender and the necessity of work are both being vigorously challenged and, in some cases, subverted (Frayne, 2015; Tudor, 2019).

Each of the broad approaches to the stratification of mental illness that we have discussed – intersectional, configurational and definitional – suggests that the mental health crisis cannot be fully addressed if the response is restricted to facilitating access to mental health services and designing public health campaigns encouraging people to 'seek help'. Rather, they underline the need to consider more deeply the economic distribution of wealth and cultural politics surrounding identities. To repeat: mental health is not (only) about mental health, it is about the general dynamics of inequalities and identities in a changing society. As such, it raises fundamental questions – what level of *interacting* economic, social and health inequalities should we 'tolerate'? What is the point of advocating greater investment in mental health services if the roots of social inequality, oppression, discrimination and misery are left intact?

Stressful times

During the twentieth century, the Western world discovered stress. Although stress may have always existed in one way or another, its contemporary form must be understood as historically contingent. The very word, 'stress', starts being used widely in English literature only in the late nineteenth century. As we discussed in Chapter 2, drawing much from Jackson's (2013) history of the concept, stress only recently became formulated as a problem in social existence and organization, with its inherent characteristics, its debilitating outcomes and possible remedies. In the UK, a Mental Health Foundation study suggests, almost 75 per cent of people declared that they were overwhelmed by stress at some point in 2017.[5] The stress paradigm, or stress process model, suggests that the 'mental health crisis' consists of the convergence of adverse social conditions, creating irrepressible pressure on individuals, a pressure not balanced with the appropriate resources, resulting in the production of a collective malaise of disproportionate scope. And, in the long run, stress may turn into mental disorders.

To identify explanatory elements of such situations, the stress model can be broken down into two questions. First, where does all this stress come from – both stress as a feeling and as an idiom of distress? Second, why are people so vulnerable to stress? Several processes can be associated with rising levels of stress in societies, for instance the 'acceleration of time' (Rosa, 2015) that came with many technological innovations and neoliberal management at the workplace; the 'culture of evaluation' submitting anyone to the constant eyes of judgement; the material struggles that especially characterize the lives of the most disadvantaged (Speed, Moncrieff and Rapley, 2014); and the emotional tensions resulting from the generalized expectation to self-control (Elias, 2000). These processes do not necessarily imply 'worsened' conditions of life; indeed, working conditions have improved in many sectors in terms of wages, working hours or safety, and so forth. They imply a reconfiguration of the social production of stress and related emotions.

In addition, we observe a nascent economy of stress due to the neoliberal turn taken by most societies in the world. Indeed, these changes carry the perceived necessity to 'cope', or to 'relax', which requires more time, more money, specific types of cultural capital, and social networks. In this economy of stress – both a literal economy and a moral one – stress acts as a common prism to understand a variety of pressures weighing on people. Several works also raise that mental health care is often permeated by neoliberal logics encouraging patients, now tellingly 'service users' or 'customers', to be the 'entrepreneur' of their own recovery (Brijnath and Antoniades, 2016; Chowdhury, 2020, p 1349), supported by a culture of 'self-care' (Russell, 2018); this leads some to understand psychiatric and psychological care as a form of maintenance for capitalism (Roberts, 2015), caring for dysfunctions in a typical form of soft power: 'the stick had been replaced by the carrot' (Cohen, 2016, p 91). As Atkinson (2020) notes, the 'supermarket model' of social resources for individual wellbeing highlights that the very meaning of wellbeing should be reassessed then as a 'technology of soft capitalism'. As the typical side effect of what is too often called 'modernity', stress and its most worrying effects are then taken care of by the mental health apparatus, the buffer of a capitalist lifestyle, realizing a self-sufficient cycle of offer and demand – a market.

In other words, in addition to considering, as per the stress paradigm, the mental health crisis as an accumulation of maladjustments between types of stress and buffering resources due to social settings, one needs to consider more broadly the historically, culturally and economically constructed framework in which mental disorders are tied to stress. We proposed two paths to go further.

On the one hand, *the social process of stress production should be understood as embedded into inequalities*. This, as sociology has long shown, mostly takes the shape of issues revolving around class, gender and race, and includes the ideologies that make people endorse full responsibility for the place they hold in their society. This leads Sweet (2018) to call for a finer account of the 'processes of neoliberal subjectivation' (p 92) whereby individuals internalize their responsibility for debts, and experience mental distress (in addition to physical health issues). The concept of 'minority stress' (Meyer, 2003) afforded useful adjustments in this direction because it situates stress in social space: racial discrimination, sexism or class contempt generate forms of stress. As with social positions, we can assume that minority stress emerges as particularly prevalent in societies where this mix of inequality, partial consciousness of their unfair nature and belief in meritocracy announces an ongoing transition of the form and intensity of domination relations; this also helps to explain why even people who benefit from these relations, those in advantaged positions, can experience *status anxiety*.

A related line of investigation attends to gender. *Stress, and reactions to stress, are embedded into gender socialization*. A common observation in existing research suggests that too much stress would provoke 'internalizing' behaviours among women and 'externalizing' behaviours among men. Following this observation, what does the mental health crisis tell us about an amplification of such reactions to stress, especially as violence is increasingly illegitimate, which modifies the traditional 'balance' of gender (Wouters, 2007)? Certainly, gender relations are changing, albeit more slowly than some might imagine, and this may well play out in terms of how stress is expressed and experienced. This might even change measures of mental health issues. For example, one of the key markers of the 'crisis' of mental health in the UK has been rising rates of self-harm and suicide among women, especially those aged 16–24 (McManus et al, 2019). The shifts in rates of identified self-harm (hospital treated) and suicides among young women may point to increased stress, or they may point to changing ways in which young women express and respond to stress. Whatever the reason, such shifts certainly call for further examination that do not uncritically reproduce binary understandings of gender (tacitly conveyed in the dichotomy between internalization and externalization) which – in some cases – may be fuelling some of the distress being experienced (Chandler and Simopouolou, 2021).

On the other hand, in addition to 'minority stresses', we showed that the *sociology, history and anthropology of emotions enable us to refine the questions raised by the stress paradigm*: from 'where does all this stress come from?' to 'how are emotions associated with mental distress socially produced'? These emotions include angst, anxiety, fear, uncertainty, sadness, suffering *and* stress (even if the proponents of the stress paradigm would present stress as a 'transversal' process). Anger was highlighted because it is the emotion of injustice, reported by many people suffering from various disorders, but also in social movements such as #metoo, Black Lives Matter or even the Yellow Jackets; in these social movements, anger tends to be discrediting, and discredit more pronounced where activists belong to stigmatized groups. We do not mean that mental illness and social movements are the same thing: we mean that culturally, anger arises in situations deemed unfair or discriminatory, which concerns many areas of social life beyond mental health and, as such, it opens alternative analytical directions. Similarly, we evoked paranoia as it particularly epitomizes how psychology runs the risk of assuming that everybody lives in the same conditions of trust: a world where we have no reason to be paranoid, which is actually the situation of a privileged minority. We could have mentioned also shame, as a core emotion in many mental disorders and situations (Chandler, 2020), or the social production of fear and, at its extremes, phobia, (Orr, 2006). Our main point is that considering the panel of possible emotions underlying mental disorders, and how each of these emotions are generated in a systemic way, unveils other routes to understanding mental disorder beyond the generic figure of 'stress': the mental health crisis might be a crisis in the social production of emotions.

Among sociological theories, the stress model is probably the closest to policy making – even the NIC reference something called 'social isolation stress disorder' (NIC, 2021, p 23). It fits with modes of calculation necessary to put 'cost-effective' measures into place. It matches conceptions of 'science' that prevail in politics and among most funding organizations. This may, at least in part, explain the success of the stress paradigm, and provides an opportunity to recall that interpretations of the mental health crisis are deeply entangled with politics, insofar as they tap into institutionalized visions of the social order.

However, in our view, acknowledging the cultural frame in which stress can be perceived as a common prism to mental distress, underscoring how this stress relates to relations of domination, and extending our horizon to emotions at large, is more promising in addressing the 'mental health crisis'. We showed that, first, this perspective enables the crisis to be contextualized: Westerners perceive stress as their main problem, and a whole economic circuit relies on such perception. Second, the experience, definition and management of stress cannot be isolated from the social positions of the 'stressed' people, which amplifies our considerations on social position. Third, while the model of stress tends to depoliticize the mental health crisis, approaching the same crisis through anger, paranoia, shame, fear, and so forth, reveals the deeper structural, political processes in which forms of emotional distress emerge and are socially produced beyond diagnosed mental disorders.

Categorizing spirals

What does the mental health crisis look like from a *labelling perspective*? At first, the mental health crisis resonates with arguments about the extension of psy-disciplines, psy-discourses and psy-professionals. There exist more and more psy-categories that people can use to characterize their problems, understand their inabilities, name their eccentricities and channel their emotions. Although many are not sufficiently funded to reach their full potential, more and more mental health services contribute to labelling people with these categories and treating them accordingly, including with confinement, drugs and legal restrictions. As previously mentioned, many governments lean strongly on these services to alleviate the calculated economic plague of mental illness (AIHW, 2021; Vigo et al, 2019). In turn, populations are prompted to identify, understand and potentially self-treat their emotional and behavioural issues as mental disorders; any help they might receive requiring them to frame it this way. This takes place in a context where the rise of the 'mass psychological culture' (Castel, 1981) and 'therapism' is argued by some to have lowered people's threshold for emotional pain and rendered them more dependent on psychological professionals and state and medical bureaucracies (Dowbiggin, 2001); a context where 'trauma' becomes a pivotal prism to explain distress (Fassin and Rechtman, 2009). Faced with this public health concern, some agencies take charge of organizing care and producing data – with, obviously, the interest of showing the gravity of the crisis.[6] These categorizations also generate stigma, which creates the perceived need for anti-stigma campaigns. In turn, the perceived need for more mental health services and professionals – to cater for alarming levels of need – leads to the establishment of more services, that further circulate psy-representations in societies, transforming visions of the human psyche in schools, in cultural productions, and even in the law (Aïdan, 2012). In the West and, increasingly, globally, we live in societies where we are all socialized to this psychologizing way of dealing with our inner tensions. This is the categorizing spiral.

These social processes realize themselves through a range of *socio-political arrangements*. But this comes with some relatively recent complexity: today, the diffusion of psy-categories cannot be reduced to the direct action of psychiatric and psychological organizations. Diagnoses, whose articulation was once a privilege of the medical profession, permeate our cultures (Brinkmann, 2016) and take on multiple shapes and practices (Jutel and Russell, 2021). As cultural objects, psy-categories then translate into the everyday material and symbolic interests of many fields and groups, while others express ongoing resistance. Activist groups developed alternative worldviews to mainstream psychiatry, such as the psychiatric survivors movement that emerged out of the civil rights movement (see one of its foundational texts, Chamberlin, 1978), or the voice hearers movement that advocates worldwide for the production of knowledge about voice-hearing by voice hearers themselves (Gardien, 2018). In all societies, local 'non-psy' ways of making sense and regulating troubles exist, among which, first and foremost, is religion. Some communities, such as African American people in the US, are more likely to seek support at church when they experience difficulties (Dempsey et al, 2016; Blank et al, 2002). Other activities – transformational rituals, sports, activism, celebrations – are likely to have significant 'therapeutic' or 'regulatory' effects on populations. All in all, the socio-political arrangements at play in the mental health crisis cannot be reduced to psy-organizations and services, and their influence, but should encompass a web of manifold actors, from advocacy groups to alternative therapies, through the various institutions that shape mental health in its broadest sense in a given territory.

Thus, while the power of psychiatry and the contingency of its seemingly neutral categories have been widely demonstrated (Kutchins and Kirk, 1997; Whitaker, 2011; Greenberg, 2013; Whooley, 2019), the institutional assemblages through which such categorizing power persists and rapidly evolves are more difficult to grasp. In relation to the political response to (and construction of) the 'mental health crisis', it is worth noting the role of high-income countries' public health literature and institutions, which stand at the forefront of this process due to their in-between position, both in academe and public policy. Especially crucial to legitimizing the psychiatric understanding of mental health in governmental organizations are notions such as 'treatment gap', which 'refers to the percentage of individuals who require treatment in a country or a defined community but do not receive it due to various reasons' (presented and criticized by Pathare et al, 2018, p 463) and 'unmet needs', a concept that can be measured with several methods, from asking participants what prevents them from using services (Christidis et al, 2018) to asking mental health professionals what publics they think should be more in contact with them (Rens et al, 2020) through comparing territories and assuming that those with lower prevalence rates are under-diagnosing potential patients (Andrews and Henderson, 2000). These concepts present it as a given that individuals who meet the criteria for mental disorders but do not seek professional help 'actually' need it without knowing it. In these measurements, non-medical forms of labelling and care, such as religious or family-based, are dismissed as inappropriate, ineffective or driven by ignorance. However, strong critiques have been levelled at medical models of care for mental health, including suicide prevention, suggesting these may in some cases deter help-seeking (Fitzpatrick and River, 2018). Thus, the mental health crisis is underlain by an ideological and material struggle revolving around the monopoly of the mental health apparatus over the legitimate designation and treatment of (almost all) human problems.

Such struggles matter all the more as the labels they partially legitimize can be performative to some extent. In other words, how categories shape the experience and identities of populations should be considered alongside the socio-political arrangements that allow their use and legitimation. Most of them deeply reconfigure people's self-concept; they are biographical disruptions, or illuminations, to take a few sociological expressions. But once purely stigmatizing, many mental health labels today are actively discussed, contested, claimed in social movements (Chamak, 2008), and the stigma they carry partially reversed, such as with autism and the neurodiversity framework (McWade et al, 2015). The contemporary use of mental health categories, en masse and with strong identity implications, might signal a certain mode of subjectivation or performativity. In addition to their social statuses, many people use the distinctive clues they perceive in their own cognitive, emotional or behavioural functioning to draw out singularities that define themselves socially. Perhaps mental disorders can now be understood *in part* as cultural practices, as Bourdieu studied them in the 1970s: they not only reflect individual sensitivities, but are also ways of positioning oneself in the social space, notably in comparison with others. Different categories of mental disorder might ultimately help people 'become someone', or rather to use the common expression, 'becoming oneself'. Taking forms of suffering as forms of identification would turn what Fassin (2011c) calls the 'compassionate ethos' to define a political attitude towards poverty, into a generalized mode of being.

CONCLUSION

Let us finally address the question: *why diagnosis? And, why labelling?* In most neoliberal universities, after going through psychological evaluation, students can ask for extensions or specific arrangements. Understanding or not, most teachers do not want to dedicate too much time to administrative tasks, so they grant most requests quite easily. So why do students still need to get an official paper attesting that they 'have something'? Similarly, a wide portion of the population that experience emotional and behavioural difficulties could decide to use alternative categories, or no category at all. But if *one* teacher refuses to grant students the extension they think they need, or if *one* executive does not understand a worker's requests to set up working arrangements, then this student can see their degree being compromised while this worker can face serious career issues. Asking for informal agreements is a risk. Here is a self-powered spiral, again: while psychiatric and psychological categories spread, they act as a legitimate justification in most administrations, and this obliges more and more people to seek them, especially in large, impersonal institutions. From this angle, the necessity of labelling can be read as a side effect of the rise of bureaucracy and neoliberal management where people have *no other excuse* not to perform; in which case the mental health crisis can be read as a form of 're-formalization' of our societies, to take Wouters' (2007) expression inspired by Elias. Further, as Grinker (2020) shows with 'the autism industrial complex' in the US, stigma reduction and the valorization of mental health-related eccentricities might be capitalized upon by many actors in neoliberal economies, from special education programmes to businesses implementing special recruitment schemes for neurodiverse workers. In sum, why humans pursue mental health labels in certain contexts cannot be reduced only to the desire of understanding their suffering, fixing their issues or refining their identities: broader institutionally and socially established modes of subjectivation arguably play a major part in the mental health crisis.

To conclude, labelling perspectives provide another light to the mental health crisis. Let us consider the plethora of psy-categories pervading societies and the socio-political arrangements that constitute and legitimize the politics of labelling. Let us review the multiple ways in which these categories then become performative. Let us take the measure of the popularity of these categories, to which people in many contemporary societies are now socialized from the earliest age. Let us observe our context where few, if any, other available and socially legitimate means exist to frame the behaviours perceived as awkward or the emotions revolving around intense suffering. All these elements combine to influence *what people become through categorizations*.

They further illuminate – but rarely do policies acknowledge these effects – how by their very existence mental health services, in caring for people diagnosed with mental disorders, shape the forms taken by these disorders.

Cultural mirrors

The World Health Organization advances the following estimations: around the world, 264 million people suffer from depression, 45 million from bipolar disorders, 20 million from schizophrenia and other psychoses. In total, this constitutes the whole population of the US, widespread throughout the earth but diagnosed with the *same* troubles. The *same* categories have been applied to all of them.

The globalization of the psychiatric model of mental illness conditions these statistics, of course, but also further paves the way for the globalization of mental health interventions. Epitomizing the global health movement, in 2019, the WHO started its 'Special Initiative for Mental Health (2019–2023): Universal Health Coverage for Mental Health'. This initiative aims 'to ensure access to quality and affordable care for mental health conditions in 12 priority countries to 100 million more people'.[7] Thereby, the universalist hypothesis, according to which mental disorders would be the same for all populations with some slight 'cultural' variations, is becoming a self-fulfilling prophecy. Although the diversity of ways of apprehending emotions and healing reported by researchers around the world is astounding, international organizations export the Western model of illness to such an extent that progressively, indeed, we observe only few fundamental differences between cultures. People are increasingly socialized to perceive Western categories as the most reasonable manners of understanding their emotions and behaviours. Thus in the very notion of a 'mental health crisis' lie these power relations constitutive of the ways in which mental disorders are socially managed and felt.

Mental health is intimately tied to colonial dynamics, and more largely to geopolitical processes. This fact has become inescapable for a twenty-first century sociologist of mental health. Seriously acknowledging these dynamics and their most intimate effects both on collective organizations and individual psyches would deeply enhance contemporary collective reflections in this field.

In particular, the influence of 'Western' representations on the issues experienced by people in 'non-Western' countries has now been convincingly demonstrated (Watters, 2010, and Katzman et al, 2004). *Cultural loss* in colonized areas is the prototypical illustration of this. But the *cultural clash* and *consonance models*, according to which individuals experience mental distress when living between two cultures, through contradictory expectations or insufficient integration, can also be interpreted through this lens. Indeed, these theorizations of a human need to 'fit in' cannot be fully understood without comprehending the political contexts that, in different fashions, underpin movements of population, the racialization of certain populations as well as the construction of migration as a social problem. The mental health crisis attends to how 'cultures' have been historically constructed as (often one-dimensional) integrative entities in which individuals can find happiness – and it denotes a collective trouble in this regard.

In this context, can we further our understanding of how cultures 'produce' mental disorders, all the more to the scope a generalized crisis? Chapter 4 reviewed the main possibilities in the literature and presented two final avenues, on which we will focus here. The first one consists of reversing the epistemological status attributed to mental illness: *thinking of 'madness' beyond the deficit narrative*. There are several ways to do so, such as seeing mental disorders as the atypical appropriation of cultural objects, the processing of traumatic history, the collective problematization of mental life, the realization of an expressive potential, or the manifestation of an ethical stance towards the world. From this standpoint, the mental health crisis could be the sign of the recomposing articulation between rationality, functionality and disability in neoliberal social organizations; heralding the diversification of people and the – both public and intimate – recognition of such diversity, as per sexual orientation and identity. The crisis would be a transitional phase in a broader democratic process towards increased tolerance of neurodiversity and everyone's touch of craziness. It would be the outcome of a greater sensitivities regarding individual inner struggles, interpersonal relations, but also environments, as per, for instance, new forms of grief and sadness associated with climate change.

The second option is to take the multiple critiques addressed to the notion of culture (as a too 'monolithic' or reductionist concept) into account and design *integrative models* that merge several aspects of social life in the production of mental health and illness. We mentioned several attempts to combine genetics, brain functioning and social processes, which raise methodological problems that would need to be solved for this approach to be helpful in understanding the mental health crisis. Hacking's theory of ecological niches happens to constitute an interesting illustration of what an integrated model would look like, as it combines parts of the four main approaches we have identified in this book: social position, stress, labelling and culture. According to this model, the mental health crisis – provided that all mental illnesses can be comprehended in this model (Brossard, 2019) – would consist of increasing rates and numbers of disorders increasingly fulfilling four 'vectors':

1. *Medical taxonomy*: the multiplication and extension of psychiatric and psychological categories makes it more likely for any human problem to find its way in a medical or psychological classification.
2. *Observability*: the introspective culture in which the massification of psy-discourses socializes us, as well as the multiplication of professionals using psychologically inspired knowledge, makes it more likely for any trouble to be observed (or self-observed).

3. *Cultural polarity*: an increasing number of people find themselves in moral ambivalences where the social figures they can find in their society do not exactly match their own situation, emotions and behaviours (this vector probably evolved with the popularization of mental illness).
4. *Evasion*: if the development of mental disorders corresponds to a desire to escape one's daily constraints, then the multiplication of mental disorders could represent the increased perceived illegitimacy of these constraints or the tightening of these constraints, making certain settings unbreathable.

Despite all these theoretical elaborations, mental health policies remain focused on the 'old' notion of culture and use it as a tool to adjust pre-established initiatives and categories to 'local settings', either in low-income countries (international help) or within national territories ('scaling up' public health interventions). The core belief of these initiatives is that small adjustments – such as reimbursing 'narrative therapy' as a special treat for indigenous people in Australia, without addressing issues surrounding sovereignty or land ownership – can correct the ethnocentric track taken by some mental health initiatives.

Culture, a concept that was once a stepping stone for the proponents of cultural relativism, became the soft power arm of (mostly Western but not only) globalization. The 'mental health crisis' both as reality and construct should be seen as a part of this process.

Towards bigger pictures

If there were one thing to remember about this book, an idea that transcends its pages, it is that that *mental health is not about mental health*. This slogan-like formula, certainly simplistic, nonetheless epitomizes that mental health concerns inequalities, identities, cultural imaginaries, discriminations, politics, categorizations, capitalism and emotions, among many other things.

As such, the specialization of mental health research and services is not necessarily a beneficial process. Not only does such specialization result in the routinization of many arguments as taken-for-granted, fostering circular reasoning and research questions (for instance, 'is schizophrenia stigmatizing' or 'does stress provoke depression'?); it also encourages the production of specialized intellectuals and practitioners whose horizons are obscured, partial. Close to Weber's 'specialists without spirit', we could become spirited specialists of the spirit *only*, methodically, endlessly refining the same connections between mental disorders taken as special orders of fact, and other expected phenomena (stress, stigma, cultural differences); missing the bigger picture.

The four axes around which we have organized our book represent an attempt to approach this bigger picture. Our point is: mental disorders, this vague array of emotions and behaviours deemed pathological, should be understood and responded to as embedded in (not only correlated with) social stratifications; thought of through the unequal production of potentially stressful emotions; considered as tied up with the politics of labelling and categorizations; and examined within the historically situated notions of culture in which they emerge.

Sociology has much to offer in understanding those experiences categorized as 'mental illness', but these conversations and reflections must move out of specialist sub-disciplines into broader and more general arenas of debate. More straightforwardly, perhaps the social sciences of mental health should simply shift into a form of general sociology. As more and more people report or identify as suffering from mental disorders, and the majority of populations will have some interaction with mental health services at least once in their lifetime, this shift becomes ever more urgent.

Beyond the sole issue of knowledge production, isolating mental health from social processes – missing the bigger picture – (as most mental health policies do) presents another risk. In the current context such isolation tends to tacitly reinforce a prevalent ideology of wellbeing, wherein mental health, balance, if not happiness, appears as an autonomous purpose in and for itself. Hence policies approach mental disorders as a problem to fix, much in the same ways damaged roads and dysfunctional electricity pylons should be quickly repaired. But why? Why should remaining 'mentally healthy' be a substantive goal for human life? If social life largely determines individual mental health, the mental health of individuals does not systematically reveal the 'health', 'functioning' or 'goodness' of their society.

In other words, behind the goal of making people healthy stands a moral appreciation of what deserves to be experienced by humans and realized by collectives. There can be no proper sociology of mental health without tackling these underlying political and moral philosophies at play in the definition of what life in society means, what is valued, what makes it 'healthy' or 'troubled'. This moral appreciation is part of the bigger picture and a last reason why the sociology of mental health could be better understood as sociology in general.

Sociologists then navigate between empathy with and support towards sufferers, and radical doubts on the 'function' of their sought-after happiness. This establishes a *complimentary but critical* discrepancy with most clinical and policy approaches, a critical complementarity that both leads us to question, for instance, how neoliberalism produces actual suffering and how this suffering is also socially constructed; how the defunding of public healthcare affects the most vulnerable fractions of the population and how this care reverberates more or less tacit forms of domination.

In sum, it questions the raison d'être of health, distress and care themselves. We can be happy in a dictatorship; we can be mentally well while destroying others and our planet; we can feel better in passively reproducing exploitative structures; relaxed in not struggling against them; we can recover from mental illness without a purpose in our lives; we can be healthy without a cause.

Notes

Introduction

1. The *Diagnostic and Statistical Manual of Mental Disorders* is published by the American Psychiatric Association since 1952. It is currently in its 5th edition (released in 2013). Alongside the International Classification of Diseases (ICD), which is managed by the World Health Organization, the DSM is one of the key documents in formalizing the content and structure of psychiatric diagnoses. Although the DSM is elaborated in the US, by the 'American' Psychiatric Association, it has a global reach and influence, even in countries (such as the UK) which formally follow the ICD classification of diseases.

Chapter 1

1. This survey has led to more than 600 publications (see www.icpsr.umich.edu/web/ICPSR/studies/6153/publications). The most exhaustive report seems to be Robins and Regier (1991).
2. The *Diagnostic and Statistical Manual of Mental Disorders* is published by the American Psychiatric Association since 1952. It is currently in its 5th edition (released in 2013). Alongside the International Classification of Diseases (ICD), which is managed by the World Health Organization, the DSM is one of the key documents in formalizing the content and structure of psychiatric diagnoses. Although the DSM is elaborated in the US, by the 'American' Psychiatric Association, it has a global reach and influence, even in countries (such as the UK) which formally follow the ICD classification of diseases.
3. There are some exceptions, such as lawyers (Koltai et al, 2018) and other high-status occupations prone to difficulties related to stress, life–work balance and burn out. Sometimes education level is *inversely* correlated with levels of mental disorders, for instance in some studies of depression (Akhtar-Danesh and Landeen, 2007).
4. In the US, all pregnant women with incomes below 133 per cent of the federal poverty level (below $15,300) can ask for this help.
5. Among the manifold works presenting these approaches, see Eaton (1980, pp 157–160); Miles (1987, Chapter 7); Fox (1990); Yu and Williams (1999); Pilgrim and Rogers (2002); Elovainio et al (2012); Jin et al (2020).
6. These reasonings are not always explicit and often tacitly combined in publications. We sought to 'isolate' them to present them in the clearest way possible, without citing specific authors.
7. To go further: on how race was progressively seen as a social construction in research, see Takeuchi and Gage (2003); and on critical race theory, black and material feminist theories, indigenous perspectives and postcolonial theories in mental health research, see Varcoe et al (2019).

8. Note that, while intersectionality exists as such as a paradigm in the academic world, 'definitional' and 'configurational' approaches are re-constructions that we operated based on our analysis of the reasonings identified in the literature.
9. See also the 'multiple-hierarchy stratification perspective' (Schieman and Plickert, 2007), the 'triple jeopardy hypothesis' (Rosenfield, 2012), the 'environmental affordances model' (Mezuk et al. 2013) or the 'multilevel analysis of individual heterogeneity and discriminatory accuracy' (Evans and Erickson, 2019).
10. Widger does not use the term 'intersectionality'; this is our analysis of his work.
11. Resembling the concepts of assemblage and network, 'configuration' designates a network of interdependent units, developed by Elias with a view of bridging the divide between 'micro' and 'macro' scales in social theory (Quintaneiro, 2006). Most works we present in this section do not use this notion; however, it will help to formulate the commonalities of their reasoning.
12. There would be much to add in view of what Pinto (2014), in her ethnography of Indian psychiatric care, calls 'ethics of dissolution'. Pinto shows that psychiatry does not only try to 'fix' family vulnerabilities (and mostly women, who are often coping the most with repercussions of family issues), but also helps its members manage the inherent instability and uncertainty of kinship – here, the entanglement between healthcare and configuration.
13. The anthology *The Colour of Madness* (Linton and Walcott, 2018) addresses the 'whitewashing' of mental health in the UK drawing on a range of academic and non-academic perspectives.
14. Our emphasis on intentionality of this mechanism might sound like an overstatement. However, we underline that much political debate surrounding welfare and border policies in the Global North *intentionally* signals to the unemployed and migrants that their life should be more difficult – thus their wellbeing more stifled – than those who have a job and who are born in those wealthy countries (and see Mills, 2018; Tyler, 2020).

Chapter 2

1. For example, in 1910 the journalists of *Ballarat Star*, a newspaper in regional Australia, attributed King Edward VII's fatal health problems to the 'stress of kingship', 'anxiety to do his duty' and 'strain and work of office'.
2. For elaborations of this typology, see Schieman (2019), Thoits (2010) and Wethington et al (2004).
3. The same debates occurred around social drift versus social causation hypotheses (Aneshensel, 1992, p 18).
4. https://books.google.com/ngrams
5. Exceptions include apparent 'paradoxes' such as dominated groups facing more adversity while reporting lower levels of distress (about African Americans, see Schwartz and Meyer, 2010), and privileged groups reporting higher level of distress, attached to their difficulty to maintain a work-life balance (Schieman et al, 2006), especially lawyers (Koltai et al, 2018) and medical professionals (Grace and VanHeuvelen, 2019).
6. This model has also been applied to other groups, such as autistic people (Botha and Frost, 2018), which suggests the possibility of a downward spiral of adverse situations producing stress, that produces disorders and labelling, that produce stress, and so forth.
7. See Chapters 1 and 4, and Alang (2016).
8. The American Sociological Association mental health section award for career achievement, which provides the winner an opportunity to take stock of this field of research in the US.

9. In the same vein, the David Lynch Foundation offers, all over the world, transcendental meditation workshops for students in high-crime areas to supposedly help them master any violent inclination.
10. Summerfield (2000) notes that most psychiatric categories are designed to account for subjects living in peace, which complicates mental health projects in countries at war.

Chapter 3

1. Goffman's intervention in mental health research is represented in his publication of *Asylums* in 1961 and *Stigma* in 1963. Despite its considerable importance, we focus less on Goffman here, as he is less concerned with how mental disorders emerge (so much as how they are responded to) and in this regard, his reflections can be subsumed in Scheff's theory, and Foucault's to a lesser extent (keeping in mind our objective is to identity *reasonings* more than tracing an exhaustive history of ideas).
2. Scheff synthesized the labelling theory of mental illness in nine points: residual transgressions come from fundamentally diverse sources (social, psychological, biological, and so forth); relative to the rate of treated mental illnesses, the rate of unrecorded residual transgressions is extremely high; most residual transgressions are standardized and have ephemeral meanings; stereotypical imagery of mental illness is learned in early childhood; the stereotypes of madness are constantly being inadvertently reaffirmed in ordinary social interactions; the so-called 'deviant' people can be rewarded for playing the stereotypical role of deviant; people labelled as deviant are punished when they try to return to conventional roles; during the crisis that occurs when a residual transgression is publicly labelled, the deviant is highly suggestible and can accept the diffuse role of insane as the only possibility; of the residual rule violators, labelling is one of the most important causes of entry into residual deviance careers.
3. This is, however, a major trend in its contemporary appropriation (Farrington and Murray, 2014; Joongyeup et al, 2014). This debate gets back to Gove's (1975) argument according to which questionnaire surveys 'show' that people do not stigmatise those designated as mentally ill; which would, according to him, 'disprove' Scheff's theory. Link et al (1989) retorted that these results tell us more about what one would be expected to say in a questionnaire than about the acts themselves.
4. Among which the multiplication of public mental health campaigns in Western countries (Lawless et al, 2014).
5. Timmermans and Tietbohl (2018, p 209) encourage medical sociologists to follow the 'strong financial rationale that drives the growing expansion of medical jurisdiction'. It is true that medicalization is often implicitly taken by sociologist as an ideological motive.
6. Pescosolido et al (2008) organized these layers into an 'integrative model of stigma'.
7. These are the preliminary results of an ongoing study conducted by Brossard.
8. Garnoussi (2007) notes the development of a 'psycho-philo-spiritual nebula' made of companies and institutions producing meanings that 'fill the gap' left by wavering religious significations of the world.
9. This point has been discussed in several directions, from Brossard (2019) who argues that no matter what kind they are, mental disorders can all be approached through Hacking's theory of ecological niches, prioritizing their social dimensions, to Tsou (2016) for whom psychiatry should focus on natural kinds.

Chapter 4

1. 'I see sociology both as a system of knowledge oriented to history and as *constituted by that history*. In this way, the displacement of racialised structures from the account of modernity

2. 'To the anthropologist, our customs and those of a New Guinea tribe are two possible social schemes for dealing with a common problem, and in so far as he (sic) remains an anthropologist he is bound to avoid any weighting of one in favor of the other.' (Benedict, 1934a, p 1) About the divide between the normal and the 'abnormal', see Benedict (1934b).

3. Schizophrenia and autism were long thought to have uniform prevalence rates; however, this hypothesis tends to be disproven even in medical and epidemiological research (on schizophrenia, McGrath et al, 2008; Luhrmann and Marrow, 2016; on autism, Chiarotti and Venerosi, 2020).

4. This Foucauldian analysis of psychotropic drugs is close to Fullagar and O'Brien (2013), on women with depression in Australia.

5. Abend (2020) recently clarified the implications of this expression.

6. This reasoning dates back to, at least, the early twentieth century, when European psychiatrists noted that foreigners were over-represented among patients diagnosed with schizophrenia (at the time *dementia praecox*), reflecting waves of migrations and political turmoil. In France, a significant proportion of people diagnosed with schizophrenia were Eastern European women in the early twentieth century, Jews in the 1930s and 1940s, and North Africans in the aftermath of the Second World War (Guillemain, 2019, pp 100–106).

7. This conclusion raises measurement issues: it is likely that people experiencing mental health problems, due to their symptoms and potential stigmatisation, feel more disaffiliated from their culture than others, reporting less 'cultural consonance'. Therefore, this finding would be more of a methodological artefact than a conclusion on the dynamics of mental health.

8. Durkheim, Freud, Marx and Weber were already worried about what 'modernity' would do to people, and the loss of collectives, or meaningful relationships, is still part of the evils of capitalism associated with mental distress by contemporary authors (Matthews, 2019).

9. The same could be said of the adjective 'social', as addressed in Brossard et al (2020).

10. A combination of Southern theory and disability studies is proposed under the name 'Southern Disability Studies' by St Guillaume and Finlay (2018).

11. This could include a sociological reconsideration of the psychological works of Vygostky (as Lignier, 2020, proposes), Meyerson or Bruner.

12. The recent special issue of *International Review of Psychiatry*, introduced by Romero et al (2020), gives a good overview of this movement in Abya Yala (Latin America).

Conclusion

1. For example, Jorm's (2018) research suggests that the 'Better Access' scheme in Australia, a policy that started in 2006 and conceptualised mental health issues as resulting from insufficient access to care, and therefore improved access to care, was not correlated by a decrease in measured severe psychological distress. This finding contrasts with others (Pirkis et al, 2011) that showed how people previously undiagnosed became diagnosed with this scheme and then reported better psychological health. This illustrates the difference between population health (not impacted by the scheme, as per Jorm) and individual responses to medical attention (measured by Pirkis et al). Since then, prevalence rates kept growing and the Australian Institute of Health and Welfare later communicated, AU$10.6 billion was spent by the federal government on mental health services in 2018–2019,

NOTES

while 4.4 million Australians (almost 1 in 5) received mental-health related prescriptions in 2019–2020. In 2021, the Australian parliament launched a series of debates to review mental health policy in the country, and preserved exactly the same reasoning, almost exclusively focused on Medicare reimbursement rates for various healthcare services.

2   www.mentalhealth.org.uk/statistics/
3   'Lifetime prevalence' means the percentage of people who will likely suffer from a disorder at some point of their life given the national average measured at a given moment.
4   www.nimh.nih.gov/health/statistics/mental-illness
5   www.mentalhealth.org.uk/statistics/
6   Hence more and more agencies, with a view to emphasising the need for more mental health services, measure not only 'depression' or 'anxiety disorder', but 'depressive symptoms' or 'anxiety' at large, which obviously makes numbers skyrocket, justifying the need for more services.
7   www.who.int/health-topics/mental-health. The WHO also offers a uniformised atlas of the mental health situation in most countries: www.who.int/publications/i/item/9789240036703

References

Abend, G. (2020) 'Making things possible', *Sociological Methods & Research*, Online first.

Abend, G., Petre, C. and Sauder, M. (2013) 'Styles of causal thought: An empirical investigation', *American Journal of Sociology*, 119(3): 602–654.

Abi-Rached, J. (2020) *Asfūriyye: A History of Madness, Modernity, and War in the Middle East*, Cambridge, MA: MIT Press.

Abraham, J. (2010) 'Pharmaceuticalization of society in context: Theoretical, empirical and health dimensions', *Sociology*, 44(4): 603–622.

Abrutyn, S. and Mueller, A. (2016) 'When too much integration and regulation hurts: Reenvisioning Durkheim's altruistic suicide', *Society and Mental Health*, 6(1): 56–71.

Abrutyn, S. and Mueller, A. (2018) 'Towards a cultural-structural theory of suicide: Examining excessive regulation and its discontents', *Sociological Theory*, 36(1): 48–66.

Adams, A., Vail, L., Buckingham, C.D., Kidd, J., Weich, S. and Roter, D. (2014) 'Investigating the influence of African American and African Caribbean race on primary care doctors' decision making about depression', *Social Science and Medicine*, 116: 161–168.

Adams, T.L. (2010) 'Gender and feminization in health care professions', *Sociology Compass*, 4: 454–465.

Adeponle, A.B., Groleau, D. and Kirmayer, L.J. (2015) 'Clinician reasoning in the use of cultural formulation to resolve uncertainty in the diagnosis of psychosis', *Culture, Medicine and Psychiatry*, 39: 16–42.

Ahmed, S. (2006) *Queer Phenomenology: Orientations, Objects, Others*, Durham, NC: Duke University Press.

Aïdan, G. (2012) 'L'invention du sujet psychique en droit', PhD dissertation, Paris: CERSA.

Ajrouch, K.J. and Antonucci, T.C. (2018) 'Social relations and health: Comparing "invisible" Arab Americans to Blacks and Whites', *Society and Mental Health*, 8(1): 84–92.

Akhtar-Danesh, N. and Landeen, J. (2007) 'Relation between depression and sociodemographic factors', *International Journal of Mental Health Systems*, 1(4): 1–9.

REFERENCES

Alang, S.M. (2016) '"Black folk don't get no severe depression": Meanings and expressions of depression in a predominantly black urban neighborhood in Midwestern United States', *Social Science and Medicine*, 157: 1–8.

Albor, C., Uphoff, E.P., Stafford, M., Ballas, D., Wilkinson, R.G. and Pickett, K.E. (2014) 'The effects of socioeconomic incongruity in the neighbourhood on social support, self-esteem and mental health in England', *Social Science and Medicine*, 111: 1–9.

Albrecht, G. (2005) 'Solastalgia: A new concept in human health and identity', *Philosophy, Activism, Nature*, 3: 41–55.

Alexander, J., Eyerman, R., Giesen, B., Smelser, N. and Sztompka, P. (eds) (2004) *Cultural Trauma and Collective Identity*, Berkeley, CA: University of California Press.

Allouch, A. (2021) *Mérite*, Paris: Anamosa.

Almedom, A.M. (2005) 'Social capital and mental health: An interdisciplinary review of primary evidence', *Social Science and Medicine*, 61(5): 943–964.

American Psychiatric Association (2013) *Diagnostic and Statistical Manual of Mental Disorders: DSM-5*, Arlington, VA: American Psychiatric Association.

Anderson, W., Jenson, D. and Keller, R. (2011) *Unconscious Dominions: Psychoanalysis, Colonial Trauma, and Global Sovereignties*, Durham, NC: Duke University Press.

Andersson, M.A. and Harkness, S.K. (2018) 'When do biological attributions of mental illness reduce stigma? Using qualitative comparative analysis to contextualize attributions', *Society and Mental Health*, 8(3): 175–194.

Andrews, G. and Henderson, S. (eds) (2000) *Unmet Need in Psychiatry: Problems, Resources, Responses*, Cambridge: Cambridge University Press.

Aneshensel, C.S. (1992) 'Social stress: Theory and research', *Annual Review of Sociology*, 18: 15–38.

Aneshensel, C.S. (2009) 'Toward explaining mental health disparities', *Journal of Health and Social Behavior*, 50: 377–394.

Aneshensel, C.S. (2015) 'Sociological inquiry into mental health: The legacy of Leonard I. Pearlin', *Journal of Health and Social Behavior*, 56: 166–178.

Aneshensel, C.S. and Avison, W.R. (2015) 'The stress process', *Society and Mental Health*, 5(2): 67–85.

Ansloos, J. and Peltier, S. (2021) 'A question of justice: critically researching suicide with Indigenous studies of affect, biosociality, and land-based relations', *Health*, DOI: 13634593211046845.

Antonakakis, N. and Collins, A. (2014) 'The impact of fiscal austerity on suicide: On the empirics of a modern Greek tragedy', *Social Science and Medicine*, 112: 39–50.

Araya, R., Dunstan, F., Playle, R., Thomas, H., Palmer, S. and Lewis, G. (2006) 'Perceptions of social capital and the built environment and mental health', *Social Science and Medicine*, 62(12): 3072–3083.

Armstrong, D. (1995) 'The rise of surveillance medicine', *Sociology of Health & Illness*, 17: 393–404.

Armstrong, D. (1997) 'Foucault and the sociology of health and illness: A prismatic reading', in R. Bunton and A. Peterson (eds) *Foucault, Health and Medicine*, London: Routledge, pp 39–55.

Atkinson, S. (2020) 'The toxic effects of subjective wellbeing and potential tonics', *Social Science & Medicine*, 288: 113098.

Australian Institute of Health and Welfare (AIHW) (2021) 'Mental health services in Australia'. Available from: www.aihw.gov.au/reports/mental-health-services/mental-health-services-in-australia [Accessed 30 November 2021]

Bacchus, D. (2008) 'Coping with work-related stress: A study of the use of coping resources among professional Black women', *Journal of Ethnic & Cultural Diversity in Social Work*, 17(1): 60–81.

Baert, S., De Visschere, S., Schoors, K., Vandenberghe, D. and Omey, E. (2016) 'First depressed, then discriminated against?', *Social Science and Medicine*, 170: 247–254.

Bains, J. (2005) 'Race, culture and psychiatry: A history of transcultural psychiatry', *History of Psychiatry*, 16(2): 139–154.

Balandier, G. (1951) 'La situation coloniale', *Cahiers Internationaux de Sociologie*, 11: 44–79.

Balandier, G. (1970) *The Sociology of Black Africa*, London: Deutsch.

Balland, L. (2020) 'Le désengagement impossible. L'angoisse des professeurs des écoles débutants', *Tracés. Revue de Sciences humaines*, 38: 83–101.

Baller, R. and Richardson, K. (2009) 'The "dark side" of the strength of weak ties: The diffusion of suicidal thoughts', *Journal of Health and Social Behavior*, 50: 261–276.

Barbee, H., Moloney, M.E. and Konrad, T.R. (2018) 'Selling slumber: American neoliberalism and the medicalization of sleeplessness', *Sociology Compass*, 12: e12622.

Barker, K. (2008) 'Electronic support groups, patient-consumers, and medicalization: The case of contested illness', *Journal of Health and Social Behavior*, 49(1): 20–36.

Barnard, A. (2019) 'Bureaucratically split personalities: (Re)Ordering the mentally disordered in the French state', *Theory and Society*, 48: 753–784.

Barnes, D. and Bates, L. (2017) 'Do racial patterns in psychological distress shed light on the Black–White depression paradox? A systematic review', *Social Psychiatry and Psychiatric Epidemiology*, 52(8): 913–928.

Barnes, D., Lieff, S., Eschliman, E., YiPing, L. and Yang, L. (2020) 'The immigrant mental health advantage in the US among ethnic minority and other groups', in G. Nagayama Hall (ed) *Mental and Behavioral Health of Immigrants in the United States*, Cambridge: Academic Press, pp 219–252.

Baron-Cohen, S. (2002) 'The extreme male brain theory of autism', *Trends in Cognitive Sciences*, 6(6): 248–254.

Barr, B., Kinderman, P. and Whitehead, M. (2015) 'Trends in mental health inequalities in England during a period of recession, austerity and welfare reform 2004 to 2013', *Social Science and Medicine*, 147: 324–331.

Barrett, A. and Turner, J. (2005) 'Family structure and mental health: The mediating effects of socioeconomic status, family process, and social stress', *Journal of Health and Social Behavior*, 46: 156–169.

Barrett, R.J. (1996) *The Psychiatric Team and the Social Definition of Schizophrenia*, Cambridge: Cambridge University Press.

Bassett, E. and Moore, S. (2013) 'Social capital and depressive symptoms: The association of psychosocial and network dimensions of social capital with depressive symptoms in Montreal, Canada', *Social Science and Medicine*, 86: 96–102.

Bateson, G. (1972) *Steps to an Ecology of Mind: Collected Essays in Anthropology, Psychiatry, Evolution, and Epistemology*, San Francisco, CA: Chandler.

Bauldry, S. (2015) 'Variation in the protective effect of higher education against depression', *Society and Mental Health*, 5(2): 145–161.

Baum, E. (2017) *The Invention of Madness: State, Society, and the Insane in Modern China*, Chicago, IL: University of Chicago Press.

Bauman, Z. (2007) *Consuming Life*, Cambridge: Polity Press.

Beam, C., Dinescu, D., Emery, R. and Turkheimer, E. (2017) 'A twin study on perceived stress, depressive symptoms, and marriage', *Journal of Health and Social Behavior*, 58(1): 37–53.

Becares, L., Nazroo, J. and Kelly, Y. (2015) 'A longitudinal examination of maternal, family, and area-level experiences of racism on children's socioemotional development: Patterns and possible explanations', *Social Science and Medicine*, 142: 128–135.

Becker, G. (1978) *The Mad Genius Controversy: A Study in the Sociology of Deviance*, Beverly Hills, CA: SAGE.

Becker, H.S. (1963) *Outsiders: Studies in the Sociology of Deviance*, New York, NY: Macmillan.

Becker, H.S. (1967) 'Whose side are we on?', *Social Problems*, 14: 239–247.

Behrouzan, O. (2015) 'Writing prozāk diaries in Tehran: Generational anomie and psychiatric subjectivities', *Culture Medicine and Psychiatry*, 39: 399–426.

Béliard, A., Eideliman, J-S., Fansten, M., Jiménez-Molina, Á., Mougel, S. and Planche, M. (2018) 'Le TDA/H, un diagnostic qui agite les familles', *Anthropologie & Santé*, 17(1): online.

Bell, A. (2014) 'Life-course and cohort trajectories of mental health in the UK, 1991–2008 – a multilevel age-period-cohort analysis', *Social Science and Medicine*, 120: 21–30.

Bendelow, G. (2009) *Health, Emotion, and the Body*, Cambridge: Polity Press.

Benedict, R. (1934a) *Patterns of Culture*, New York, NY: Houghton Mifflin Harcourt.

Benedict, R. (1934b) 'Anthropology and the abnormal', *Journal of General Psychology*, 10: 59–82.

Bergmans, R.S. and Wegryn-Jones, R. (2020) 'Examining associations of food insecurity with major depression among older adults in the wake of the Great Recession', *Social Science and Medicine*, 258: 113033.

Beshai, S., Mishra, S., Meadows, T., Parmar, P. and Huang, V. (2017) 'Minding the gap: Subjective relative deprivation and depressive symptoms', *Social Science and Medicine*, 173: 18–25.

Best, J. (2001) 'Social progress and social problems: Toward a sociology of gloom', *The Sociological Quarterly*, 42(1): 1–12.

Bhambra, G.K. (2014) 'A sociological dilemma: Race, segregation and US sociology', *Current Sociology*, 62: 472–492.

Bhambra, G.K. (2016) 'Postcolonial reflections on sociology', *Sociology*, 50: 960–966.

Bhambra, G.K. and Holmwood, J. (2021) *Colonialism and Modern Social Theory*, Cambridge: Polity Press.

Bierman, A. (2014) 'Reconsidering the relationship between age and financial strain among older adults', *Society and Mental Health*, 4(3): 197–214.

Billaud, J. (2012) 'Suicidal performances: Voicing discontent in a girls' dormitory in Kabul', *Culture, Medicine and Psychiatry*, 36: 264–285.

Blackdog Institute (2020) 'Facts & figures about mental health'. Available from: www.blackdoginstitute.org.au/wp-content/uploads/2020/04/1-facts_figures.pdf [Accessed 30 November 2021]

Blank, M., Mahmood, M., Fox, J. and Guterbock, T. (2002) 'Alternative mental health services: The role of the Black Church in the South', *American Journal of Public Health*, 92: 1668–1672.

Blaxter, M. (1978) 'Diagnosis as category and process: The case of alcoholism', *Social Science and Medicine*, 12: 9–17.

Blazer, D. (2005) *The Age of Melancholy: 'Major Depression' and Its Social Origins*, London: Routledge.

Blum, P., Minoc, J. and Weber, F. (2015) 'Familles en danger? Psychiatrie, hébergement familial et vulnérabilité', *Informations sociales*, 188: 68–75.

Bonnin, J.E. (2017) 'Formulations in psychotherapy: Admission interviews and the conversational construction of diagnosis', *Qualitative Health Research*, 27(11): 1591–1599.

Bonnin, J.E. (2020) *Discourse and Mental Health: Voice, Inequality and Resistance in Medical Settings*. London: Routledge.

REFERENCES

Bonnington, O. and Rose, D. (2014) 'Exploring stigmatisation among people diagnosed with either bipolar disorder or borderline personality disorder: A critical realist analysis', *Social Science and Medicine*, 123: 7–17.

Botha, M. and Frost, D.M. (2018) 'Extending the minority stress model to understand mental health problems experienced by the autistic population', *Society and Mental Health*, 10(1): 20–34.

Bourdieu, P. (1979) *La Distinction*, Paris: Minuit.

Bourdieu, P. (1980) *Le Sens Pratique*, Paris: Minuit

Bourgois, P. (1995) *In Search of Respect: Selling Crack in El Barrio*, Cambridge: Cambridge University Press.

Bowers, L. (1998) *The Social Nature of Mental Illness*, London: Routledge.

Bowleg, L. (2008) 'When Black + lesbian + woman ≠ Black lesbian woman: The Methodological challenges of qualitative and quantitative intersectionality research', *Sex Roles*, 59(56): 312–325.

Bowleg, L. and Bauer, G. (2016) 'Invited reflection: Quantifying intersectionality', *Psychology of Women Quarterly*, 40(3): 337–341.

Bracke, P., Pattyn, E. and Von Dem Knesebeck, O. (2013) 'Overeducation and depressive symptoms: Diminishing mental health returns to education', *Sociology of Health & Illness*, 35(8): 1242–1259.

Bracke, P., Delaruelle, K., Dereuddre, R. and Van de Velde, S. (2020) 'Depression in women and men, cumulative disadvantage and gender inequality in 29 European countries', *Social Science and Medicine*, 267: 113354.

Braedley, S. (2012) 'The masculinization effect: Neoliberalism, the medical paradigm and Ontario's health care policy', *Canadian Women's Studies/Cahier des Femmes*, 29(3): 71–83.

Bridger, E. and Daly, M. (2020) 'Intergenerational social mobility predicts midlife well-being: Prospective evidence from two large British cohorts', *Social Science and Medicine*, 261: 113217.

Brijnath, B. and Antoniades, J. (2016) '"I'm running my depression": Self-management of depression in neoliberal Australia', *Social Science and Medicine*, 152: 1–8.

Brinkmann, S. (2016) *Diagnostic Cultures: A Cultural Approach to the Pathologization of Modern Life*, Farnham: Ashgate.

Bröer, C. and Besseling, B. (2017) 'Sadness or depression: Making sense of low mood and the medicalization of everyday life', *Social Sciences and Medicine*, 183: 28–36

Bromberg, W. (1942) 'Some social aspects of the history of psychiatry', *Bulletin of the History of Medicine*, 11: 117–132.

Brooks, B.B. (2014) 'Chucaque and social stress among Peruvian highlanders', *Medical Anthropology Quarterly*, 28(3): 419–439.

Brossard, B. (2014) 'Fighting with oneself to maintain the interaction order: A sociological approach to self-injury daily process', *Symbolic Interaction*, 37: 558–575.

Brossard, B. (2018) *Why Do We Hurt Ourselves? Understanding Self Harm in Social Life*, Bloomington, IN: Indiana University Press.

Brossard, B. (2019) 'Why mental disorders flourish and wither: Extending the theory of ecological niches', *Social Science and Medicine*, 237: 112445.

Brossard, B. and Sallée, N. (2020) 'Sociology and psychology: What intersections?', *European Journal of Social Theory*, 23(1): 3–14.

Brossard, B. and Weber, F. (2016) '"Folie et société": ce qu'apporte et ce que manque la question du handicap', in V. Boucherat-Hue, D. Leguay, B. Pachoud, A. Plagnol and F. Weber (eds) *Handicap Psychique: Questions Vives*, Toulouse: Erès, pp 173–191.

Brossard, B., Cruwys, T., Zhou, H. and Helleren-Simpson, G. (2020) 'What do we mean by "social" in mental health research?', *Social Science and Medicine*, 261: 113233.

Brown, P. (1995) 'Naming and framing: The Social construction of diagnosis and illness', *Journal of Health and Social Behavior*, (extra issue): 34–52.

Brown, R.L., Richman, J., Moody, M. and Rospenda, K. (2018) 'The enduring mental health effects of post-9/11 discrimination in the context of the Great Recession: Race/Ethnic variation', *Society and Mental Health*, 9(2): 158–170.

Brown, T.N., Donato, K.M., Laske, M.T. and Duncan, E.M. (2013) 'Race, nativity, ethnicity, and cultural influences in the sociology of mental health', in C.S. Aneshensel, J. Phelan and A. Bierman (eds) *Handbook of the Sociology of Mental Health*, New York, NY: Springer, pp 255–276.

Burgard, S.A. and Seelye, S. (2017) 'Histories of perceived job insecurity and psychological distress among older U.S. adults', *Society and Mental Health*, 7(1): 21–35.

Busfield, J. (1996) *Men, Women and Madness: Understanding Gender and Mental Disorder*, London: Macmillan.

Busfield, J. (2014) 'Gender and mental illness', in W.C. Cockerham, R. Dingwall and S. Quah (eds) *The Wiley Blackwell Encyclopedia of Health, Illness, Behavior, and Society*, Chichester: Wiley, pp 620–629.

Busfield, J. (2017) 'The concept of medicalisation reassessed', *Sociology of Health and Illness*, 39: 759–774.

Butterworth, P., Gill, S., Rodgers, B., Anstey, K., Willamil, E. and Melzer, D. (2006) 'Retirement and mental health: analysis of the Australian national survey of mental health and well-being', *Social Science and Medicine*, 62(5): 1179–1191.

Button, M. and Marsh, I. (eds) (2020) *Suicide and Social Justice: New Perspectives on the Politics of Suicide and Suicide Prevention*, London: Routledge.

Cairns, J.M., Graham, E. and Bambra, C. (2017) 'Area-level socioeconomic disadvantage and suicidal behaviour in Europe: A systematic review', *Social Science and Medicine*, 192: 102–111.

Callard, F. and Fitzgerald, D. (2015) *Rethinking Interdisciplinarity across the Social Sciences and Neurosciences*, Basingstoke: Palgrave Macmillan.

Camp, D., Finlay, W.M.L. and Lyons, E. (2002) 'Is low self-esteem an inevitable consequence of stigma? An example from women with chronic mental health problems', *Social Science & Medicine*, 55: 823–834.

Campbell, D. (2021) 'Extent of mental health crisis in England at "terrifying" level', *The Guardian*, 9 April. Available from: www.theguardian.com/uk-news/2021/apr/09/extent-of-mental-health-crisis-in-england-at-terrifying-level [Accessed 30 November 2021]

Canguilhem, G. (1991 [1943]) *The Normal and the Pathological*, Princeton, NJ: Princeton University Press.

Cant, S. (2017) 'Hysteresis, social congestion and debt: towards a sociology of mental health disorders in undergraduates', *Social Theory & Health*, 16(4): 311–325.

Carde, E. (2021) 'Les inégalités sociales de santé au prisme de l'intersectionnalité', *Sciences sociales et santé*, 39: 5–30.

Carpenter-Song, E. (2009) 'Caught in the psychiatric net: meanings and experiences of ADHD, pediatric bipolar disorder and mental health treatment among a diverse group of families in the United States', *Culture, Medicine and Psychiatry*, 33(1): 61–85.

Carter, R., Shimkets, R.P. and Bornemann, T.H. (2014) 'Creating and changing public policy to reduce the stigma of mental illness', *Psychological Science in the Public Interest*, 15(2), 35–36.

Castel, F., Castel, R. and Lovell, A. (1982) *The Psychiatric Society*, New York, NY: Columbia University Press.

Castel, P.-E. (2012) *La Fin des Coupables*, Paris: Ithaque.

Castel, R. (1981) *La Gestion des Risques. De L'antipsychiatrie à L'après-pychanalyse*, Paris: Minuit.

Castel, R. (1988) *The Regulation of Madness: The Origins of Incarceration in France*, Berkeley, CA: California University Press.

Chamak, B. (2008) 'Autism and social movements: French parents' associations and international autistic individuals' organisations', *Sociology of Health & Illness*, 30: 76–96.

Chamak, B. and Bonniau, B. (2013) 'Changes in the diagnosis of autism: How parents and professionals act and react in France', *Culture, Medicine and Psychiatry*, 37: 405–426.

Chamberlin, J. (1978) *On Our Own: Patient Controlled Alternatives to the Mental Health System*, New York, NY: Haworth Press.

Chan, T.W. (2018) 'Social mobility and the well-being of individuals', *British Journal of Sociology*, 69(1): 183–206.

Chandler, A. (2016) *Self-Injury, Medicine and Society: Authentic Bodies*, Basingstoke: Palgrave Macmillan.

Chandler, A. (2018) 'Seeking secrecy: A qualitative study of younger adolescents' accounts of self-harm, *YOUNG: Nordic Journal of Youth Research*, 26: 313–331.

Chandler, A. (2019) 'Boys don't cry? Critical phenomenology, self-harm and suicide', *The Sociological Review*, 67(6): 1350–1366.

Chandler, A. (2020) 'Shame as affective injustice: Qualitative, sociological explorations of self-harm, suicide and socioeconomic inequalities', in M. Button and I. Marsh (eds) *Suicide and Social Justice*, London: Routledge, pp 32–49.

Chandler, A. and Simopoulou, Z. (2021) 'The violence of the cut: Gendering self-harm', *International Journal of Environmental Research and Public Health*, 18(9):46–50.

Chandler, A., Myers, F., and Platt, S. (2011) 'The construction of self-injury in the clinical literature: A sociological exploration' *Suicide and Life Threatening Behavior*, 41, 1, 98–109.

Chartonas, D. and Bose, R. (2015) 'Fighting with spirits: Migration trauma, acculturative stress, and new sibling transition – A Clinical case study of an 8-year-old girl with absence epilepsy', *Culture, Medicine and Psychiatry*, 39(4): 698–724.

Cheslack-Postava, K. and Jordan-Young, R.M. (2012) 'Autism spectrum disorders: Toward a gendered embodiment model', *Social Science and Medicine*, 74(11): 1667–1674.

Chevance, A., Clément, J. and Weber, F. (2021) 'Présentations' in M. Mauss (ed) *Sociologie, Psychologie, Physiologie*, Paris: PUF.

Chiarotti, F. and Venerosi, A. (2020) 'Epidemiology of autism spectrum disorders: A Review Of Worldwide Prevalence Estimates Since 2014', *Brain Sciences*, 10(5): 274.

Chowdhury, N. (2020) 'Practicing the ideal depressed self: Young professional women's accounts of managing depression', *Qualitative Health Research*, 30(9): 1349–1361.

Christidis, P., Lin, L. and Stamm, K. (2018) 'An unmet need for mental health services', *Monitor on Psychology*, 49(4): 19.

Chua, J.L. (2012) 'The register of "complaint"', *Medical Anthropology Quarterly*, 26: 221–240.

Clarke, A.E., Shim, J.K., Mamo, L., Fosket, J.R. and Fishman, J.R. (2003) 'Biomedicalization: Technoscientific transformations of health, illness, and U.S. biomedicine', *American Sociological Review*, 68(2): 161–194.

Cluver, L., Shenderovich, Y., Meinck, F., Berezin, M.N., Doubt, J. and Ward, C.L. (2020) 'Parenting, mental health and economic pathways to prevention of violence against children in South Africa', *Social Science and Medicine*, 262: 113194.

Cobb, M.C. (2018) 'Casualties of debate: A critique of the sociology of emotion', *Sociology Compass*, 12: e12643.

Coe, G. (2021) 'Decolonising mental illness', *Australian Journal of Social Issues*, Online first.

Coelho, P. (1998) *Veronika Decides to Die*, New York, NY: Harper Collins.

Cohen, B. (2014) 'Passive-aggressive: Māori resistance and the continuance of colonial psychiatry in Aotearoa New Zealand', *Disability and the Global South*, 1(2): 319–339.

Cohen, B. (2016) *Psychiatric Hegemony: A Marxist Theory of Mental Illness*, London: Palgrave Macmillan.

Cohn, B. (1996) *Colonialism and Its Forms of Knowledge: The British in India*. Princeton, NJ: Princeton University Press.

Collin, J. and David, P.-M. (eds) (2016) *Vers une Pharmaceuticalisation de la Société? Le Médicament Comme Objet Social*, Québec: Presses de l'université du Québec.

Collins, P.H. (2015) 'Intersectionality's definitional dilemmas', *Annual Review of Sociology*, 41(1): 1–20.

Collins, P.H. and Bilge, S. (2016) *Intersectionality*, Chichester: Wiley.

Collins, P.Y., von Unger, E., Armbrister, A. (2008) 'Church ladies, good girls, and locas: Stigma and the intersection of gender, ethnicity, mental illness, and sexuality in relation to HIV risk', *Social Science and Medicine*, 67(3): 389–397.

Comaroff, J. and Comaroff, J. (1987) 'The madman and the migrant: Work and labor in the historical consciousness of a South African people', *American Ethnologist*, 14(2): 191–209.

Conrad, P. (2007) *The Medicalization of Society*, Baltimore, MD: John Hopkins University Press.

Conrad, P. and Potter, D. (2000) 'From hyperactive children to ADHD adults: Observations on the expansion of medical categories', *Social Problems*, 47(4): 559–582.

Conrad, P. and Schneider, J. (1980) *Deviance and Medicalization: From Badness to Sickness*, Philadelphia, PA: Temple University Press.

Cook, B., Doksum, T., Chen, C-N., Carle, A. and Alegria, M. (2013) 'The role of provider supply and organization in reducing racial/ethnic disparities in mental health care in the U.S.', *Social Science and Medicine*, 84: 102–109.

Coope, C., Gunnell, D., Hollingworth, W., Hawton, K., Kapur, N., Fearn, V., Wells, C. and Metcalfe, C. (2014) 'Suicide and the 2008 economic recession: Who is most at risk? Trends in suicide rates in England and Wales 2001–2011', *Social Science and Medicine*, 117: 76–85.

Cooper, D. (1971) *The Death of the Family*, New York, NY: Penguin.

Cooper, D. (1978) *The Language of Madness*, New York, NY: Penguin.

Cooper, F. (2004) 'Development, modernization, and the social sciences in the era of decolonization: The examples of British and French Africa', *Revue d'Histoire des Sciences Humaines*, 1(1): 9–38.

Cooper, K. (2020) 'Are poor parents poor parents? The relationship between poverty and parenting among mothers in the UK', *Sociology*, 55(2): 349–383.

Corrigan, P. and Fong, M. (2014) 'Competing perspectives on erasing the stigma of illness: What says the dodo bird?', *Social Science and Medicine*, 103: 110–117.

Corrigan, P. and Watson, A. (2002) 'Understanding the impact of stigma on people with mental illness', *World Psychiatry*, 1(1):16–20.

Coutant, I. and Eideliman, J.S. (2013) 'The moral economy of contemporary working-class adolescence: Managing symbolic capital in a French public "Adolescent Centre"', *British Journal of Sociology*, 64(2): 248–266.

Cover, R. (2012) *Queer Youth Suicide, Culture and Identity: Unliveable Lives?* London: Routledge.

Crenshaw, K. (1991) 'Mapping the Margins: Intersectionality, Identity Politics, and Violence against Women of Color', *Stanford Law Review*, 43(6): 1241–99.

Cresswell, M. (2005) 'Psychiatric "survivors" and testimonies of self-harm', *Social Science and Medicine*, 61(8): 1668–1677.

Crossley, N. (1998) 'R. D. Laing and the British anti-psychiatry movement: A socio-historical analysis', *Social Science & Medicine*, 47(7): 877–889.

Cruwys, T., Haslam, S., Dingle, G., Haslam, C. and Jetten, J. (2014) 'Depression and social identity: An integrative review', *Personality and Social Psychology Review*, 18(3): 215–238.

Cunsolo, A. and Ellis, N.R. (2018) 'Ecological grief as a mental health response to climate change-related loss', *Nature Climate Change*, 8: 275–281.

Curtis, C. and Curtis, B. (2011) 'The origins of a New Zealand suicidal cohort: 1970–2007', *Health Sociology Review*, 20(2): 219–228.

Curtis, S., Pearce, J., Cherrie, M., Dibben, C., Cunningham, N. and Bambra, C. (2019) 'Changing labour market conditions during the 'great recession' and mental health in Scotland 2007–2011: An example using the Scottish Longitudinal Study and data for local areas in Scotland', *Social Science and Medicine*, 227: 1–9.

Damaske, S., Smyth, J. and Zawadzki, M. (2014) 'Has work replaced home as a haven? Re-examining Arlie Hochschild's Time Bind proposition with objective stress data', *Social Science and Medicine*, 115: 130–138.

Darin-Mattsson, A., Andel, R., Celeste, R.K. and Kareholt, I. (2018) 'Linking financial hardship throughout the life-course with psychological distress in old age: Sensitive period, accumulation of risks, and chain of risks hypotheses', *Social Science & Medicine*, 201: 111–119.

Darmon, M. (2017) *Becoming Anorectic: A Sociological Study*, London: Routledge.

Davies, J. (2021) *Sedated: How Modern Capitalism Created Our Mental Health Crisis*, London: Atlantic Books

Davis, N. (1972) 'Labeling theory in deviance research: A critique and reconsideration', *The Sociological Quarterly*, 13(4): 447–474.

de Boise, S. and Hearn, J. (2017) 'Are men getting more emotional? Critical sociological perspectives on men, masculinities and emotions', *The Sociological Review*, 65(4): 779–796.

De Gaulejac, V. (1987) *La Névrose de Classe*, Paris: Ellen Corin.

De Moortel, D., Palència, L., Artazcoz, L., Borrell, C. and Vanroelen, C. (2015) 'Neo-Marxian social class inequalities in the mental well-being of employed men and women: the role of European welfare regimes', *Social Science & Medicine*, 128: 188–200.

Deleuze, G. (2013) *Pourparlers*, Paris: Minuit.

Delille, E. and Crozier, I. (2018) 'Historicizing transcultural psychiatry: People, epistemic objects, networks, and practices', *History of Psychiatry*, 29(3): 257–262.

del Mar García-Calvente, M., Hidalgo, N., Del Rio Lozano, M., Marcos Marcos, J., Martínez-Morante, E. and Maroto-Navarro, G. (2012) 'Exhausted women, tough men: A qualitative study on gender differences in health, vulnerability and coping with illness in Spain', *Sociology of Health & Illness*, 34(6): 911–926.

Dempsey, K., Butler, S.K. and Gaither, L. (2016) 'Black Churches and mental health professionals: Can this collaboration work?', *Journal of Black Studies*, 47(1): 73–87.

Dengah, H., Bingham, I., Thomas, E., Hawvermale, E. and Temple, E. (2019) '"Find that balance": The impact of cultural consonance and dissonance on mental health among Utah and Mormon Women', *Medical Anthropology Quarterly*, 33: 439–458.

Denneson, L., Tompkins, K., McDonald, K., Hoffmire, C., Britton, P., Carlson, K., Smolenski, D. and Dobscha, S. (2020) 'Gender differences in the development of suicidal behavior among United States military veterans: A national qualitative study', *Social Science & Medicine*, 260: 113178.

Derek Cheung, Y., Spittal, M., Williamson, M., Tung, S. and Pirkis, J. (2014) 'Predictors of suicides occurring within suicide clusters in Australia, 2004–2008', *Social Science & Medicine*, 118: 135–142.

Devereux, G. (1939) 'A sociological theory of schizophrenia', *Psychoanalytic Review*, 26: 315–342.

Devereux, G. (1980) *Basic Problems in Ethnopsychiatry*, Chicago, IL: University of Chicago Press.

Dinos, S., Stevens, S., Serfaty, M., Weich, S. and King, M. (2004) 'Stigma: The feelings and experiences of 46 people with mental illness: Qualitative study', *British Journal of Psychiatry*, 184(2): 176–181.

Dixon, J. (2015) 'Treatment, deterrence or labelling: Mentally disordered offenders' perspectives on social control', *Sociology of Health & Illness*, 37: 1299–1313.

Dohrenwend, B. (2000) 'The role of adversity and stress in psychopathology: Some evidence and its implications for theory and research', *Journal of Health and Social Behavior*, 41(1): 1–19.

Donovan, R. and West, L. (2014) 'Stress and mental health: Moderating role of the strong Black woman stereotype', *Journal of Black Psychology*, 41(4): 384–396.

Dostoevsky, F. (1998[1879]) *Brothers Karamazov*, Grand Rapids, MI: Christian Classics Ethereal Library.

Dowbiggin, I. (2011) *The Quest for Mental Health: A Tale of Science, Medicine, Scandal, Sorrow, and Mass Society*, New York, NY: Cambridge University Press.

Dressler, W., Balieiro, M. and Santos, J. (1998) 'Culture, socioeconomic status, and physical and mental health in Brazil', *Medical Anthropology Quarterly*, 12: 424–446.

Dressler, W., Balieiro, M., Ribeiro, R. and Dos Santos J. (2007) 'Cultural consonance and psychological distress: Examining the associations in multiple cultural domains', *Culture Medicine and Psychiatry*, 31(2):195–224.

Dressler, W., Balieiro, M., Ferreira de Araújo, L, Silva, W. and Ernesto Dos Santos, J. (2016) 'Culture as a mediator of gene-environment interaction: Cultural consonance, childhood adversity, a 2A serotonin receptor polymorphism, and depression in urban Brazil', *Social Science and Medicine*, 161: 109–17.

Du Bois, W.E.B. (2007) *The Philadelphia Negro: A Social Study*, Oxford University Press.

Dudgeon, P. and Walker, R. (2015) 'Decolonising Australian psychology: Discourses, strategies, and practice', *Journal of Social and Political Psychology*, 3(1): 276–297.

Duncan, W. (2015) 'Transnational disorders: Returned migrants at Oaxaca's psychiatric hospital', *Medical Anthropology Quarterly*, 29: 24–41.

Durkheim, E. (1952 [1897]) *Suicide: A Study in Sociology*, London: Routledge & Kegan Paul.

Eaton, W. (1980) *The Sociology of Mental Disorders*, New York, NY: Praeger.

Eggerman, M. and Panter-Brick, C. (2010) 'Suffering, hope, and entrapment: resilience and cultural values in Afghanistan', *Social Science & Medicine*, 71(1): 71–83.

Ehrenberg, A. (2010) *The Weariness of Self: Diagnosing the History of Depression in the Contemporary Age*, Montreal: McGill-Queen's University Press.

Ekman I. (2016) 'Beyond medicalization: Self-injuring acts revisited', *Health*, 20(4): 346–362.

Elias, N. (2000 [1939]) *The Civilizing Process*, London: Blackwell.

Elovainio, M., Pulkki-Råback, L., Jokela, M., Kivimäki, M., Hintsa, T., Viikari, J., Raitakari, O. and Keltikangas-Järvinen, L. (2012) 'Socioeconomic status and the development of depressive symptoms from childhood to adulthood: A longitudinal analysis across 27 years of follow-up in the Young Finns study', *Social Science and Medicine*, 74(6): 923–929.

Emerson, R. (2015) *Everyday Troubles: The Micro-Politics of Interpersonal Conflict*, Chicago, IL: University of Chicago Press

Emerson, R. and Messinger, S. (1977) 'The micro-politics of trouble', *Social Problems*, 25(2): 121–134.

English, D., Carter, J., Bowleg, L., Malebranche, D., Talan, A. and Rendina, H. (2020) 'Intersectional social control: The roles of incarceration and police discrimination in psychological and HIV-related outcomes for Black sexual minority men', *Social Science and Medicine*, 258: 113121.

Enjolras, F. (2016) *Santé Mentale et Adolescence: Entre Psychiatrie et Sciences Sociales*, Nimes: Champs Social.

Ensel, W.M. and Lin, N. (1991) 'The life stress paradigm and psychological distress', *Journal of Health and Social Behavior*, 32: 321–341.

Erving, C. and Thomas, C. (2017) 'Race, emotional reliance, and mental health', *Society and Mental Health*, 8(1): 69–83.

Evans, C. and Erickson, N. (2019) 'Intersectionality and depression in adolescence and early adulthood: A MAIHDA analysis of the national longitudinal study of adolescent to adult health, 1995–2008', *Social Science and Medicine*, 220: 1–11.

Evans-Lacko, S., Corker, E., Williams, P., Henderson, C. and Thornicroft, G. (2014) 'Effect of the Time to Change anti-stigma campaign on trends in mental-illness-related public stigma among the English population in 2003–13', *The Lancet Psychiatry*, 1(2): 121–128.

Everett, B. (2015) 'Sexual orientation identity change and depressive symptoms: A longitudinal analysis', *Journal of Health and Social Behavior*, 56(1): 37–58.

Eyal, G. (2013) 'For a sociology of expertise: The social origins of the autism epidemic', *American Journal of Sociology*, 118(4): 863–907.

Eyal, G., Hart, B., Oncular, E., Oren, N. and Rossi, N. (2010) *The Autism Matrix: The Social Origins of the Autism Epidemic*, Cambridge: Polity Press.

Eyerman, R. (2001) *Cultural Trauma: Slavery and the Formation of African American Identity*, Cambridge: Cambridge University Press.

Fanon, F. (1967) *Toward the African Revolution: Political Essays*, New York, NY: Grove Press.

Fanon, F. (2019 [1952]) *Black Skins, White Masks*, New York, NY: Grove Press.

Faris, R. and Dunham, H. (1939) *Mental Disorders in Urban Areas: An Ecological Study of Schizophrenia and Other Psychoses*, Chicago, IL: University of Chicago Press.

Farrington, D. and Murray, J. (2014) *Labeling Theory: Empirical Tests*, New Brunswick, NJ: Transaction Publishers.

Fassin, D. (2004) *Des Maux Indicibles. Sociologie des Lieux Écoute*, Paris: La Découverte.

Fassin, D. and Rechtman, R. (2009) *The Empire of Trauma. An Inquiry into the Condition of Victimhood*, Princeton, NJ: Princeton University Press.

Fassin, D. (2011a) 'Racialization' in F. Mascia-Lees (ed) *A Companion to the Anthropology of the Body and Embodiment*, Chichester: Wiley, pp 419–434.

Fassin, D. (2011b) 'Policing borders, producing boundaries. The governmentality of immigration in dark times', *Annual Review of Anthropology*, 40(2): 213–226.

Fassin, D. (2011c) *The Humanitarian Reason. A Moral History of the Present*, Berkeley, CA: University of California Press.

Fassin, D. (2021) 'Of plots and men: The heuristics of conspiracy theories', *Current Anthropology*, 62(2): 128–137.

Fekete, L. (2020) 'Coercion and compliance: The politics of the "hostile environment"', *Race & Class*, 62: 97–109.

Fernández, A.T. and Gutierrez, M.C. (2020) 'Colonialism, gender and mental health in psychology: A view from Eastern Cuba', *International Review of Psychiatry*, 32(4): 340–347.

Fernandez, M., Breen, L. and Simpson, T. (2014) 'Renegotiating identities: Experiences of loss and recovery for women with bipolar disorder', *Qualitative Health Research*, 24(7): 890–900.

Fernando, S. (2017) *Institutional Racism in Psychiatry and Clinical Psychology*, Basingstoke: Palgrave Macmillan.

Ferrazzi, P. and Krupa, T. (2016) '"Symptoms of something all around us": Mental health, Inuit culture, and criminal justice in Arctic communities in Nunavut, Canada', *Social Science and Medicine*, 165: 159–167.

Feyeux, A. (2021) 'La fabrique psychiatrique (des troubles) du genre', *Sociétés Contemporaines*, 121(1): 111–138.

Fisher, M. (2011) 'The privatisation of stress', *Soundings*, 48: 123–133.

Fitzgerald, D., Rose, N. and Singh, I. (2016a) 'Living well in the neuropolis', *The Sociological Review*, 64: 221–237.

Fitzgerald, D., Rose, N. and Singh, I. (2016b) 'Revitalizing sociology: Urban life and mental illness between history and the present', *British Journal of Sociology*, 67: 138–160.

Fitzpatrick, M. (2017) *Invisible Scars: Mental Trauma and the Korean War*, Vancouver: UBC Press.

Fitzpatrick, S. and River, J. (2018) 'Beyond the medical model: Future directions for suicide intervention services', *International Journal of Health Services*, 48(1): 189–203.

Flore, J. (2020) *A Genealogy of Appetite in the Sexual Sciences*, Cham: Palgrave.

Fong, V. (2011) *Paradise Redefined: Transnational Chinese Students and the Quest for Flexible Citizenship in the Developed World*, Palo Alto, CA: Stanford University Press.

Fothergill, K., Ensminger, M., Doherty, E., Juon, H. and Green, K. (2016) 'Pathways from early childhood adversity to later adult drug use and psychological distress: A prospective study of a cohort of African Americans', *Journal of Health and Social Behavior*, 57: 223–239.

Foucault, M. (2006 [1961]) *History of Madness*, New York, NY: Routledge.

Foucault, M. (1973 [1963]) *The Birth of the Clinic*, New York, NY: Pantheon Books.

Foucault, M. (1970 [1966]) *The Order of Things*, London: Tavistok.

Foucault, M. (2002 [1969]) *The Archaeology of Knowledge*, London: Routledge.

Foucault, M. (1977 [1975]) *Discipline and Punish*, New York, NY: Random.

Foucault, M. (1979 [1976]) *The History of Sexuality Volume 1*, London: Allen Lane.

Fox, J. (1990) 'Social class, mental illness, and social mobility: The social selection-drift hypothesis for serious mental illness', *Journal of Health and Social Behavior*, 31(4): 344–353.

Francis, A. (2015) *Family Trouble: Middle-Class Parents, Children's Problems, and the Disruption of Everyday Life*, New Brunswick, NJ: Rutgers University Press.

Fraser, S., Pienaar, K., Dilkes-Frayne, E., Moore, D., Kokanovic, R., Treloar, C. and Dunlop, A. (2017) 'Addiction stigma and the biopolitics of liberal modernity: A qualitative analysis', *International Journal of Drug Policy*, 44: 192–201.

Frayne, D. (2015) *The Refusal of Work: The Theory and Practice of Resistance to Work*, London: Zed Books

Freidson, E. (1970) *Profession of medicine: A study of the sociology of applied knowledge*, New York, NY: Harper & Row

Freund, P. (2010) 'Embodying psychosocial health inequalities: Bringing back materiality and bioagency', *Social Theory & Health*, 9(1): 59–70.

Friberg, T. (2009) 'Burnout: From Popular culture to psychiatric diagnosis in Sweden', *Cult Med Psychiatry*, 33: 538–558.

Friedman, J. (2009) 'The "social case"', *Medical Anthropology Quarterly*, 23: 375–396.

Friedman, S. (2015) 'Habitus clivé and the emotional imprint of social mobility', *The Sociological Review*, 64(1): 129–147.

Frieh, E. (2020) 'Stigma, trauma and sexuality: The experiences of women hospitalised with serious mental illness', *Sociology of Health & Illness*, 42(3): 526–543.

Frost, D., LeBlanc, A., deVries, B., Alston-Stepnitz, E., Stephenson, R. and Woodyatt, C. (2017) 'Couple-level minority stress: An examination of same-sex couples' unique experiences', *Journal of Health and Social Behavior*, 58(4): 455–472.

Fullagar, S. and O'Brien, W. (2013) 'Problematizing the neurochemical subject of anti-depressant treatment: The limits of biomedical responses to women's emotional distress', *Health*, 17(1): 57–74.

Gardien, E. (2018) 'De l'utilité des groupes de pairs pour produire des savoirs fondés sur l'expérience: l'exemple des entendeurs de voix', *Participations*, 3(22): 29–51.

Garnoussi, N. (2007) 'De nouvelles propositions de sens pratique dans le domaine de l'existentiel', PhD Dissertation, Paris: EPHE.

Gibson, P. (2014) 'Gender and self-salience', in W.C. Cockerham, R. Dingwall and S. Quah (eds) *The Wiley Blackwell Encyclopedia of Health, Illness, Behavior, and Society*, Chichester: Wiley.

Giddens, A. (1991) *Modernity and Self-Identity: Self and Society in the Late Modern Age*, Cambridge: Polity Press.

Giles, D. (2014) 'DSM-V is taking away our identity': The reaction of the online community to the proposed changes in the diagnosis of Asperger's disorder', *Health*, 18(2): 179–95.

Giles, D. and Newbold, J. (2011) 'Self- and other-diagnosis in user-led mental health online communities', *Qualitative Health Research*, 21(3): 419–28.

Giraldi, T. (2017) *Unhappiness, Sadness and 'Depression'*, Cham: Palgrave.

Goffman, E. (1961) *Asylums: Essays on the Social Situation of Mental Patients and Other Inmates*, New York, NY: Doubleday.

Goffman, E. (1963) *Stigma: Notes on the Management of Spoiled Identity*. London: Penguin.

Goldstein, M. (1979) 'The sociology of mental health and illness', *Annual Review of Sociology*, 5(1): 381–409.

Gone, J. (2013) 'Redressing First Nations historical trauma: Theorizing mechanisms for indigenous culture as mental health treatment', *Transcultural Psychiatry*, 50: 683–706.

Gorman, R. and LeFrançois, B. (2017) 'Mad studies', in B. Cohen (ed) *Routledge International Handbook of Critical Mental Health*, Abingdon: Routledge.

Gove, W. (1975) 'The labelling theory of mental illness: A reply to Scheff', *American Sociological Review*, 40(2): 242–248.

Gove, W. (1976) 'Reply to Imershein and Simons (1976) and Scheff (1975)', *American Sociological Review*, 41(3): 564–567.

Gove, W. and Tudor, J. (1973) 'Adult sex roles and mental illness', *American Journal of Sociology*, 78(4): 812–835.

Grace, M. and VanHeuvelen, J. (2019) 'Occupational variation in burnout among medical staff: Evidence for the stress of higher status', *Social Science and Medicine*, 232: 199–208.

Graeber, D. (2004) *Fragments of an Anarchist Anthropology*, Chicago, IL: Prickly Paradigm Press.

Granek, L., Nakash, O., Ariad, S., Shapira, S. and Ben-David, M. (2020) 'The role of culture/ethnicity in communicating with cancer patients about mental health distress and suicidality', *Culture, Medicine and Psychiatry*, 44(2): 214–229.

Gray, D. (2002) '"Everybody just freezes. Everybody is just embarrassed": Felt and enacted stigma among parents of children with high functioning autism', *Sociology of Health & Illness*, 24(6): 734–749.

Greenberg, G. (2013) *The Book of Woe: The DSM and the Unmaking of Psychiatry*, New York, NY: New Rider.

Greenfeld, L. (2013) *Mind, Modernity, Madness: The Impact of Culture on Human Experience*, Cambridge, MA: Harvard University Press.

Grinker, R. (2020) 'Autism, "stigma," disability: A shifting historical terrain', *Current Anthropology*, 61(21): 55–67.

Grossi, E., Tavano Blessi, G., Sacco, P. (2019) 'Magic moments: Determinants of stress relief and subjective wellbeing from visiting a cultural heritage site', *Culture, Medicine, and Psychiatry*, 43(1): 4–24.

Guan, W. and Kamo, Y. (2016) 'Contextualizing depressive contagion: A multilevel network approach', *Society and Mental Health*, 6(2), 129–145.

Guerin, B. (2021) *Turning Mental Health into Social Action*, London: Routledge.

Guillemain, H. (2019) *Schizophrènes au XXème Siècle*, Paris: Alma.

Gulbas, L. and Zayas, L. (2015) 'Examining the interplay among family, culture, and latina teen suicidal behavior', *Qualitative Health Research*, 25(5): 689–699.

Gutierrez-Vazquez, E., Flippen, C. and Parrado, E. (2018) 'Migration and depression: A cross-national comparison of Mexicans in sending communities and Durham, NC', *Social Science and Medicine*, 219: 1–10.

Hacking, I. (1995a) *Rewriting the Soul: Multiple Personality and the Sciences of Memory*, Princeton, NJ: Princeton University Press.

Hacking, I. (1995b) 'The looping effects of human kinds', in D. Sperber, D. Premack and A. James Premack (eds) *Causal Cognition: A Multi-Disciplinary Debate*, Oxford: Clarendon, pp. 351–394.

Hacking, I. (1998) *Mad Travelers: Reflections on the Reality of Transient Mental Illnesses*, Cambridge, MA: Harvard University Press.

Hacking, I. (1999) *The Social Construction of What?* Cambridge, MA: Harvard University Press.

Hacking, I. (2004) 'Between Michel Foucault and Erving Goffman: Between discourse in the abstract and face-to-face interaction', *Economy and Society*, 33(3): 277–302.

Haggett, A. (2015) *A History of Male Psychological Disorders in Britain, 1945–1980*, Basingstoke: Palgrave.

Halfmann, D. (2019) 'Political institutions and the comparative medicalization of abortion', *Journal of Health and Social Behavior*, 60(2): 138–152.

Halfmann, D. (2011) 'Recognizing medicalization and demedicalization: Discourses, practices, and identities', *Health*. 16(2): 186–207.

Han, B.-C. (2015) *The Burnout Society*, Stanford, CA: Stanford University Press.

Hansen, A-M. (2009) 'Une histoire du spleen français au XVIIIe siècle: la transmission, évolution et naturalisation d'un fait anglais', MA Thesis, Montréal: McGill University.

Harper, D. (2011) 'Social inequality and the diagnosis of paranoia', *Health Sociology Review*, 20(4): 423–436.

Harper, D. and Speed, E. (2014) 'Uncovering recovery: The resistible rise of recovery and resilience' in E. Speed, J. Moncrieff and M. Rapley (eds) *De-Medicalizing Misery* II, London: Palgrave Macmillan, pp 40–57.

Hayes, J., McCabe, R., Ford, T., Parker, D. and Russell, G. (2021) '"Not at the diagnosis point": Dealing with contradiction in autism assessment teams', *Social Science and Medicine*, 268:113462.

Hayward, P. and Bright, J. (1997) 'Stigma and mental illness: A review and critique', *Journal of Mental Health*, 6(4): 345–354.

Hendry, N. (2017) 'Everyday anxieties: young women, mental illness and social media practices of visibility and connection', PhD dissertation, Melbourne: RMIT.

Hernández-Wolfe, P. (2011) 'Decolonization and 'mental' health: A Mestiza's journey in the Borderlands', *Women & Therapy*, 34(3): 293–306.

Herron, R., Ahmadu, M., Allan, J., Waddell, C. and Roger, K. (2020) '"Talk about it": Changing masculinities and mental health in rural places?', *Social Science and Medicine*, 258: 113099.

Hill, T. and Needham, B. (2013) 'Rethinking gender and mental health: A critical analysis of three propositions', *Social Science and Medicine*, 92: 83–91.

Hinshaw, S. (2007) *The Mark of Shame: Stigma of Mental Illness and an Agenda for Change*, Oxford: Oxford University Press.

Hirshbein, L. (2009) *American Melancholy: Constructions of Depression in the Twentieth Century*, New Brunswick, NJ: Rutgers University Press.

Hjelm, L., Handa, S., de Hoop, J., Palermo, T., Zambia CGP and MCP Evaluation Teams (2017) 'Poverty and perceived stress: Evidence from two unconditional cash transfer programs in Zambia', *Social Science and Medicine*, 177: 110–117.

Hoggart, R. (1957) *The Uses of Literacy: Aspects of Working Class Life*, London: Chatto and Windus.

Hollin, G. and Pilnick, A. (2018) 'The categorisation of resistance: Interpreting failure to follow a proposed line of action in the diagnosis of autism amongst young adults', *Sociology of Health & Illness*, 40: 1215–1232.

Hollingshead, A. and Redlich, F. (1958) *Social Class and Mental Illness: a Community Study*, New York, NY: Wiley.

Holloway, S. and Pimlott-Wilson, H. (2014) 'Enriching children, institutionalizing childhood? Geographies of play, extracurricular activities, and parenting in England', *Annals of the Association of American Geographers*, 104: 613–627.

Holman, D. (2014) '"What help can you get talking to somebody?" Explaining class differences in the use of talking treatments', *Sociology of Health & Illness*, 36: 531–548.

Holmes, M. (2004) 'Feeling beyond rules: Politicizing the sociology of emotion and anger in feminist politics', *European Journal of Social Theory*, 7: 209–227.

Horn, J. (2020) 'Decolonising emotional well-being and mental health in development: African feminist innovations', *Gender & Development*, 28(1): 85–98.

Horwitz, A. (1982) 'Sex-role expectations, power, and psychological distress', *Sex Roles*, 8: 607–623.

Horwitz, A. (2002) *Creating Mental Illness*, Chicago, IL: University of Chicago Press.

Horwitz, A. (2007) 'Distinguishing distress from disorder as psychological outcomes of stressful social arrangements', *Health*, 11(3): 273–289.

Horwitz, A. (2011) 'Creating an age of depression: The social construction and consequences of the major depression diagnosis', *Society and Mental Health*, 1(1): 41–54.

Horwitz, A. (2016) *What's Normal: Reconciling Biology and Culture*, Oxford: Oxford University Press.

Hsieh, N. (2014) 'Explaining the mental health disparity by sexual orientation', *Society and Mental Health*, 4(2): 129–146.

Huang, X., Western, M., Bian, Y., Li, Y., Côté, R. and Huang, Y. (2018) 'Social networks and subjective wellbeing in Australia: New evidence from a national survey', *Sociology*, 53(2): 401–421.

Ignatow, G. (2012) 'Mauss's lectures to psychologists: A case for holistic sociology', *Journal of Classical Sociology*, 12: 3–21.

Illich, I. (1974) *Medical Nemesis*, London: Calder & Boyars.

Ingram, R. (2016) 'Doing Mad Studies: Making (non)sense together', *Intersectionalities*, 5(3): online.

Irvine, J. (1995) 'Reinventing perversion: Sex addiction and cultural anxieties', *Journal of the History of Sexuality*, 5: 429–50.

Jackson, M. (2013) *The Age of Stress: Science and the Search for Stability*, Oxford: Oxford University Press.

Jacobs, M. and Spillman, L. (2005) 'Cultural sociology at the crossroads of the discipline', *Poetics*, 33: 1–14.

Jaworski, K. (2010) 'The gender-ing of suicide', *Australian Feminist Studies*, 25(63): 47–61.

Jaworski, K. (2014) *The Gender of Suicide*, Aldershot: Ashgate.

Jenkins, J. (2015) *Extraordinary Conditions: Culture and Experience of Mental Illness*, Berkeley, CA: University of California Press.

Jenkins, J. and Barrett, R. (eds) (2003) *Schizophrenia, Culture, and Subjectivity: The Edge of Experience*, Cambridge: Cambridge University Press.

Jenkins, J. and Carpenter-Song, E. (2008) 'Stigma despite recovery: Strategies for living in the aftermath of psychosis', *Medical Anthropology Quarterly*, 22(4): 381–409.

Jenkins, J. and Csordas, T. (2020) *Troubled in the Land of Enchantment: Adolescent Experience of Psychiatric Treatment*, Berkeley, CA: University of California Press.

Jin, Y., Dawei, Z. and He, P. (2020) 'Social causation or social selection? The longitudinal interrelationship between poverty and depressive symptoms in China', *Social Science and Medicine*, 249: 112848.

John, D., de Castro, A.B., Martin, D., Duran, B. and Takeuchi, D. (2012) 'Does an immigrant health paradox exist among Asian Americans? Associations of nativity and occupational class with self-rated health and mental disorders', *Social Science and Medicine*, 75(12): 2085–2098.

Johnson, A. (2019) 'Rejecting, reframing, and reintroducing: Trans people's strategic engagement with the medicalisation of gender dysphoria', *Sociology of Health & Illness*, 41: 517–532.

Joongyeup, L., Menard, S. and Bouffard, L. (2014) 'Extending interactional theory: The labeling dimension', *Deviant Behavior*, 35(1): 1–19.

Jorm, A. (2018) 'Australia's "Better Access" scheme: Has it had an impact on population mental health?', *Australian and New Zealand Journal of Psychiatry*, 52(11): 1057–1062.

Joseph, J. (2013) 'The use of the classical twin method in the social and behavioral sciences: The fallacy continues', *The Journal of Mind and Behavior*, 34: 1–39.

Jutel, A. (2009) 'Sociology of diagnosis: A preliminary review', *Sociology of Health & Illness*, 31: 278–299.

Jutel, A. and Nettleton, S. (2011) 'Towards a sociology of diagnosis: Reflections and opportunities', *Social Science & Medicine*, 73: 793–800.

Jutel, A. and Russell, G. (2021) 'Past, present and imaginary: Pathography in all its forms', *Health*, Online first.

Kaiser, B. and Kohrt, B. (2019) 'Why psychiatry needs the anthropologist: A reflection on 80 years of culture in mental health', *Psychiatry*, 82(3): 205–215.

Kaiser, B., Haroz, E., Kohrt, B., Bolton, P., Bass, J. and Hinton, D. (2015) '"Thinking too much": A systematic review of a common idiom of distress', *Social Science and Medicine*, 147: 170–83.

Kaiser, N., Näckter, S. and Karlsson, M. (2015) 'Experiences of being a young female Sami reindeer herder: A qualitative study from the perspective of mental health and intersectionality', *Journal of Northern Studies*, 9(2): 55–72.

Kamerade, D., Wang, S., Burchell, B., Balderson, S. and Coutts, A. (2019) 'A shorter working week for everyone: How much paid work is needed for mental health and well-being?', *Social Science and Medicine*, 241: 112353.

Kangmennaang, J. and Elliott, S. (2018) 'Towards an integrated framework for understanding the links between inequalities and wellbeing of places in low and middle income countries', *Social Science and Medicine*, 213: 45–53.

Kapp, S., Gillespie-Lynch, K., Sherman, L. and Hutman, T. (2013) 'Deficit, difference, or both? Autism and neurodiversity', *Developmental Psychology*, 49(1): 59–71.

Katzman, M., Hermans, K., Van Hoeken, D. and Hoek, H. (2004) 'Not your "typical island woman": anorexia nervosa is reported only in subcultures in Curacao', *Culture, Medicine and Psychiatry*, 28: 463–492.

Kaufman, J. (ed) (2014) *Creativity and Mental Illness*, Cambridge: Cambridge University Press

Keane, H. (2004) 'Disorders of desire: Addiction and problems of intimacy', *Journal of Medical Humanities*, 25(3): 189–204.

Kelly, K. (2014) 'The spread of "Post Abortion Syndrome" as social diagnosis', *Social Science & Medicine*, 102: 18–25.

Kessler, R. and McLeod, J. (1984) 'Sex differences in vulnerability to undesirable life events', *American Sociological Review*, 49(5): 620–631.

Kessler, R. and Neighbors, H. (1986) 'A new perspective on the relationships among race, social class, and psychological distress', *Journal of Health and Social Behavior*, 27(2): 107–115.

Kidron, C. and Kirmayer, L. (2019) 'Global mental health and idioms of distress: The paradox of culture-sensitive pathologization of distress in Cambodia', *Culture Medicine and Psychiatry*, 43(2): 211–235.

Killingsworth, B., Kokanovic, R., Tran, H. and Dowrick, C. (2010) 'A care-full diagnosis: Three Vietnamese Australian women and their accounts of becoming "mentally ill"', *Medical Anthropology Quarterly*, 24: 108–123.

Kim, M.H., Jung-Choi, K., Jun, H.J. and Kawachi, I. (2010) 'Socioeconomic inequalities in suicidal ideation, parasuicides, and completed suicides in South Korea', *Social Science and* Medicine, 70(8): 1254–1261.

King, M. and Bearman, P. (2011) 'Socioeconomic status and the increased prevalence of autism in California', *American Sociological Review*, 76(2): 320–346.

King, M., Semlyen, J., Tai, S., Killaspy, H., Osborn, D., Poelyuk, D. and Nazareth, I. (2008) 'A systematic review of mental disorder, suicide, and deliberate self harm in lesbian, gay and bisexual people', *BMC Psychiatry*, 8(70): 1–17.

Kirkpatrick, M. (2004) 'The feminization of psychiatry? Some ruminations', *The Journal of the American Academy of Psychoanalysis and Dynamic Psychiatry*, 32(1): 201–212.

Kirmayer, L., Gomez-Carrillo, A. and Veissiere, S. (2017) 'Culture and depression in global mental health: An ecosocial approach to the phenomenology of psychiatric disorders', *Social Science and Medicine*, 183: 163–168.

Kitanaka, J. (2008) 'Diagnosing suicides of resolve: Psychiatric practice in contemporary Japan', *Culture, Medicine, and Psychiatry*, 32: 152–176.

Kleinman, A. (1977) 'Depression, somatization and the "new cross-cultural psychiatry"', *Social Science and Medicine*, 11(1): 3–9.

Kleinman, A. (1991) *Rethinking Psychiatry: From Cultural Category to Personal Experience*, New York, NY: Free Press.

Kleinman, A. (1997) 'Triumph or pyrrhic victory? The inclusion of culture in DSM-IV', *Harvard Review of Psychiatry*, 4(6): 343–344.

Knifton, L. (2012) 'Understanding and addressing the stigma of mental illness with ethnic minority communities', *Health Sociology Review*, 21(3): 287–298.

Koehne, K., Hamilton, B., Sands, N. and Humphreys, C. (2013) 'Working around a contested diagnosis: Borderline personality disorder in adolescence', *Health*, 17(1): 37–56.

Kohn, M. (1973) 'Social class and schizophrenia: A critical review and a reformulation', *Schizophrenia Bulletin*, 1(7): 60–79

Kohrt, B. and Bourey, C. (2016) 'Culture and comorbidity: Intimate partner violence as a common risk factor for maternal mental illness and reproductive health problems among former child soldiers in Nepal', *Medical Anthropology Quarterly*, 30(4): 515–535.

Kohrt, B., Turner, E., Rai, S., Bhardwaj, A., Sikkema, K., Adelekun, A., Dhakal, M., Luitel, N., Lund, C., Patel, V. and Jordans, M. (2020) 'Reducing mental illness stigma in healthcare settings: Proof of concept for a social contact intervention to address what matters most for primary care providers', *Social Science and Medicine*, 250: 112852.

Kokanovic, R., Bendelow, G. and Philip, B. (2013) 'Depression: The ambivalence of diagnosis', *Sociology of Health & Illness*, 35(3): 377–90.

Koltai, J., Schieman, S. and Dinovitzer, R. (2018) 'The status-health paradox: Organizational context, stress exposure, and well-being in the legal profession', *Journal of Health and Social Behavior*, 59(1): 20–37.

Kroll-Smith, S. (2003) 'Popular media and "excessive daytime sleepiness": a study of rhetorical authority in medical sociology', *Sociology of Health & Illness*, 25(6): 625–643.

Kroska, A., Harkness, S., Thomas, L. and Brown, R. (2014) 'Illness labels and social distance', *Society and Mental Health*, 4(3): 215–234.

Krupchanka, D., Chrtková, D., Vítková, M., Munzel, D., Čihařová, M., Růžičková, T., Winkler, P., Janoušková, M., Albanese, E. and Sartorius, N. (2018) 'Experience of stigma and discrimination in families of persons with schizophrenia in the Czech Republic', *Social Science and Medicine*, 212: 129–135.

Kunz-Ebrecht, S., Kirschbaumb, C. and Steptoea, A. (2004) 'Work stress, socioeconomic status and neuroendocrine activation over the working day', *Social Science & Medicine*, 58(8): 1523–1530.

Kusserow, A. (1999) 'Crossing the great divide: Anthropological theories of the Western self', *Journal of Anthropological Research*, 55(4): 541–562.

Kutchins, H. and Kirk, S. (1997) *Making Us Crazy: DSM, the Psychiatric Bible and the Creation of Mental Disorders*, New York, NY: Free Press.

Kyaga, S. (2015) *Creativity and Mental Illness: The Mad Genius in Question*, London: Palgrave.

Kysar-Moon, A. (2019) 'Childhood adversity and internalizing problems: Evidence of a race mental health paradox', *Society and Mental Health*, 10(2): 136–162.

Kyung-Sook, W., Sangsoo, S., Sangjin, S. and Young-Jeon, S. (2018) 'Marital status integration and suicide: A meta-analysis and meta-regression', *Social Science and Medicine*, 197: 116–126.

Lahire, B. (2020) 'Sociology at the individual level, psychologies and neurosciences', *European Journal of Social Theory*, 23(1): 52–71.

Landstedt, E., Almquist, Y., Eriksson, M. and Hammarström, A. (2016), 'Disentangling the directions of associations between structural social capital and mental health: Longitudinal analyses of gender, civic engagement and depressive symptoms', *Social Science and Medicine*, 163: 135–143.

Lane, R. (2020) 'Expanding boundaries in psychiatry: uncertainty in the context of diagnosis-seeking and negotiation', *Sociology of Health and Illness*, 42: 69–83.

Lareau, A. (2002) 'Invisible inequality: Social class and childrearing in Black families and white families', *American Sociological Review*, 67: 747–776.

Larson, J. and Corrigan, P. (2008) 'The stigma of families with mental illness', *Academic Psychiatry*, 32: 87–91.

Laurence, J. (2019) 'Community disadvantage, inequalities in adolescent subjective well-being, and local social relations: The role of positive and negative social interactions', *Social Science and Medicine*, 237: 112442.

Lawless, A., Coveney, J., and MacDougall, C. (2014) 'Infant mental health promotion and the discourse of risk', *Sociology of Health & Illness*, 36: 416–431.

Lee, M. (2009) 'Neighborhood residential segregation and mental health: A multilevel analysis on Hispanic Americans in Chicago', *Social Science and Medicine*, 68(11): 1975–1984.

Lee, M. and Kawachi, I. (2017) 'The company you keep: Is socialising with higher-status people bad for mental health?', *Sociology of Health & Illness*, 39(7): 1206–1226.

Lee, S., Chiu, M., Tsang, A., Chui, H. and Kleinman, A. (2006) 'Stigmatizing experience and structural discrimination associated with the treatment of schizophrenia in Hong Kong', *Social Science and Medicine*, 62(7): 1685–1696.

Lei, X., Sun, X., Strauss, J., Zhang, P. and Zhao, Y. (2014) 'Depressive symptoms and SES among the mid-aged and elderly in China', *Social Science & Medicine*, 120: 224–232.

Leighton, A. and Hughes, J. (1961) 'Cultures as a causative of mental disorder', *The Milbank Memorial Fund Quarterly*, 39(3), 1–22.

Lemert, E. (1951) *Social Pathology: A Systematic Approach to the Theory or Sociopathic Behavior*, New York, NY: McGraw-Hill.

Lemert, E. (1962) 'Paranoia and the dynamics of exclusion', *Sociometry*, 25(1): 2–20.

Lester, R. (2004) 'Commentary: Eating disorders and the problem of 'culture' in acculturation', *Culture, Medicine and Psychiatry*, 28(4): 607–15.

Lester, R. (2007) 'Critical therapeutics: Cultural politics and clinical reality in two eating disorder treatment centers', *Medical Anthropology Quarterly*, 21(4): 369–387.

Leuenberger, C. (2006) 'Constructions of the Berlin Wall: How material culture is used in psychological theory', *Social Problems*, 53(1): 18–37.

LeVine, P. and Matsuda, Y. (2003) 'Reformulation of diagnosis with attention to cultural dynamics: Case of a Japanese woman hospitalized in Melbourne, Australia', *Culture, Medicine, and Psychiatry*, 27: 221–243.

Lévi-Strauss, C. (1949) 'L'efficacité symbolique', *Revue de l'histoire des religions*, 135(1): 5–27.

Levy, R. (1976) 'Psychosomatic symptoms and women's protest: Two types of reaction to structural strain in the family', *Journal of Health and Social Behavior*, 17: 121–133.

Lewis, D. (1973) 'Anthropology and colonialism', *Current Anthropology*, 14(5): 581–602.

Li, J. and Liu, Z. (2018) 'Housing stress and mental health of migrant populations in urban China', *Cities*, 81: 172–179.

Lignier, W. (2020) 'Words also make us: Enhancing the sociology of embodiment with cultural psychology', *European Journal of Social Theory*, 23(1):15–32.

Lima, J., Caughy, M., Nettles, S. and O'Campo, P. (2010) 'Effects of cumulative risk on behavioral and psychological well-being in first grade: Moderation by neighborhood context', *Social Science and Medicine*, 71(8): 1447–1454.

Lindström, M. and Rosvall, M. (2012) 'Marital status, social capital, economic stress, and mental health: A population-based study', *The Social Science Journal*, 49(3): 339–342.

Link, B.G. and Phelan, J. (1995) 'Social Conditions As Fundamental Causes of Disease', *Journal of Health and Social Behavior*, 80–94.

Link, B. and Phelan, J. (2001) 'Conceptualizing stigma', *Annual Review of Sociology*, 27: 363–385.

Link, B., Cullen, F., Struening, E., Shrout, P. and Dohrenwend, B. (1989) 'A modified labeling theory approach to mental disorders: An empirical assessment', *American Sociological Review*, 54(3): 400–423.

Linstrum, E. (2016) *Ruling Minds: Psychology in the British Empire*, Cambridge, MA: Harvard University Press.

Linton, L. and Walcott, R. (2018) *The Colour Of Madness*, London: Housmans.

Lippi-Green, R. (2012) *English with an Accent: Language, Ideology, and Discrimination in the United States*, New York, NY: Routledge.

Lipset, S. and Bendix, R. (1959) *Social Mobility in Industrial Society*, Berkeley, CA: University of California Press.

Littlewood, R. (2001) *Pathologies of the West: The Anthropology of Mental Illness in Euro-America*, London: Bloomsbury.

Littlewood, R. (2004) 'Commentary: Globalization, culture, body image, and eating disorders', *Culture, Medicine, and Psychiatry*, 28(4): 597–60.

Littlewood, R. and Dein, S. (2013) 'Did Christianity lead to schizophrenia? Psychosis, psychology and self reference', *Transcultural Psychiatry*, 50(3): 397–420.

Liu, K., King, M. and Bearman, P. (2010) 'Social influence and the autism epidemic', *American Journal of Sociology*, 115(5): 1387–1434.

Livingston, J. and Boyd, J. (2010) 'Correlates and consequences of internalized stigma for people living with mental illness: a systematic review and meta-analysis', *Social Science and Medicine*, 71(12): 2150–2161.

Longest, K. and Thoits, P. (2012) 'Gender, the stress process, and health', *Society and Mental Health*, 2(3): 187–206.

Louie, P. (2019) 'Revisiting the cost of skin color: Discrimination, mastery, and mental health among Black adolescents', *Society and Mental Health*, 10(1): 1–19.

Lowe, J. and DeVerteuil, G. (2020) 'Power, powerlessness and the politics of mobility: Reconsidering mental health geographies', *Social Science and Medicine*, 252: 112918.

Lu, Y. (2012) 'Household migration, social support, and psychosocial health: The perspective from migrant-sending areas', *Social Science and Medicine*, 74(2): 135–142.

Luhrmann, T. (2000) *Of Two Minds: The Growing Disorder in American Psychiatry*, New York, NY: Alfred A. Knopf.

Luhrmann, T. (2007) 'Social defeat and the culture of chronicity: Or, why schizophrenia does so well over there and so badly here', *Culture, Medicine, and Psychiatry*, 31: 135–172.

Luhrmann, T. (2020) 'Mind and spirit: A comparative theory about representation of mind and the experience of spirit', *Journal of the Royal Anthropological Institute*, 26: 9–27.

Luhrmann, T. and Marrow, J. (eds) (2016) *Our Most Troubling Madness - Case Studies in Schizophrenia Across Cultures*, Berkeley, CA: University of California Press.

Luhrmann, T., Padmavati, R., Tharoor, H. and Osei, A. (2015) 'Hearing voices in different cultures: A social kindling hypothesis', *Topics in Cognitive Science*, 7: 646–663.

Lundberg, J., Kristenson, M. and Starrin, B. (2009) 'Status incongruence revisited: Associations with shame and mental wellbeing', *Sociology of Health & Illness*, 31(4): 478–493.

Lupton, D. (1998) *The Emotional Self: A Sociocultural Exploration*, London: Sage.

Lutz, C. (1988) *Unnatural Emotions: Everyday Sentiments on a Micronesian Atoll and Their Challenge to Western Theory*, Chicago, IL: University of Chicago Press.

Macdonald, R., Shildrick, T. and Furlong, A. (2013) 'In search of "intergenerational cultures of worklessness": Hunting the Yeti and shooting zombies', *Critical Social Policy*, 34: 199–220.

Mallard, G. (2018) 'The gift as colonial ideology? Marcel Mauss and the solidarist colonial policy in the interwar era', *Journal of International Political Theory*, 14(2): 183–202.

Maltseva, K. (2018) 'Internalized cultural models, congruity with cultural standards, and mental health', *Journal of Cross-Cultural Psychology*, 49(8): 1302–1319.

Manago, B. (2015) 'Understanding the social norms, attitudes, beliefs, and behaviors towards mental illness in the United States', *Proceedings of the National Academy of Sciences*. Available from: https://sites.nationalacademies.org/cs/groups/dbassesite/documents/webpage/dbasse_170042.pdf [Accessed 30 November 2021].

Mandelbaum, J., Moore, S., Silveira, P., Meaney, M., Levitan, R. and Dubé, L. (2020) 'Does social capital moderate the association between children's emotional overeating and parental stress? A cross-sectional study of the stress-buffering hypothesis in a sample of mother-child dyads', *Social Science and Medicine*, 257: 112082.

Mann, A., Patel, T., Elbogen, E., Calhoun, P., Kimbrel, N. and Wilson, S. (2020) 'Sexual orientation, attraction and risk for deliberate self-harm: Findings from a nationally representative sample', *Psychiatry Research*, 286: 112863.

Marchand, A., Demers, A. and Durand, P. (2005) 'Does work really cause distress? The contribution of occupational structure and work organization to the experience of psychological distress', *Social Science and Medicine*, 61(1): 1–14.

Marcuse, H. (1974) *Eros and Civilization: A Philosophical Inquiry into Freud*, Boston, MA: Beacon Press.

Marcussen, K., Gallagher, M. and Ritter, C. (2019) 'Mental illness as a stigmatized identity', *Society and Mental Health*, 9(2): 211–227.

Marsh, I. (2010) *Suicide: Foucault, History and Truth*, Cambridge: Cambridge University Press.

Martin, E. (2007) *Bipolar Expeditions: Mania and Depression in American Culture*, Princeton, NJ: Princeton University Press.

Matías-Carrelo, L., Chávez, L., Negrón, G., Canono, G., Aguilar-Gaxiola, S. and Hoppe, S. (2003) 'The Spanish translation and cultural adaptation of five mental health outcome measures', *Culture, Medicine, and Psychiatry*, 27: 291–313.

Matthews, D. (2019) 'Capitalism and mental health', *Monthly Review*, 70(8): online.

Maturo, F. and Moretti, V. (2018) *Digital Health and the Gamification of Life*, Bingley: Emerald.

Mauss, M. (1921) 'L'expression obligatoire des sentiments', *Journal de psychologie*, 18: 425–434.

Mauss, M. (1926) 'Effet physique chez l'individu de l'idée de mort suggérée par la collectivité' [The physical effect on the individual of the idea of death suggested by the collectivity], *Journal de Psychologie Normale et Pathologique*, 23: 653–669.

Mauss, M. (1979) *Sociology and Psychology*, London: Routledge.

Maxfield, A. (2020) 'Testing the theoretical similarities between food and water insecurity: Buffering hypothesis and effects on mental wellbeing', *Social Science and Medicine*, 244: 112412.

Maynard, D. and Turowetz, J. (2019) 'Doing abstraction: Autism, diagnosis, and social theory', *Sociological Theory*, 37(1): 89–116.

McCulloch, J. (1995) *Colonial Psychiatry and the African Mind*, Cambridge: Cambridge University Press.

McDade, T. (2002) 'Status incongruity in Samoan youth: A biocultural analysis of culture change, stress, and immune function', *Medical Anthropology Quarterly*, 16(2): 123–50.

McDermott, E. and Roen, K. (2016) *Queer Youth, Suicide and Self-Harm – Troubled Subjects, Troubling Norms*, Basingstoke: Palgrave Macmillan.

McEwen, C. and McEwen, B. (2017) 'Social structure, adversity, toxic stress, and intergenerational poverty: An early childhood model', *Annual Review of Sociology*, 43: 445–472.

McGann, P., Hutson, D. and Katz Rothman, B. (eds) (2011) *Sociology of Diagnosis*, Bingley: Emerald.

McGinty, E., Goldman, H., Pescosolido, B. and Colleen, B. (2015) 'Portraying mental illness and drug addiction as treatable health conditions: Effects of a randomized experiment on stigma and discrimination', *Social Science and Medicine*, 126: 73–85.

McGrath, J., Saha, S., Chant, D. and Welham, J. (2008) 'Schizophrenia: A concise overview of incidence, prevalence, and mortality', *Epidemiological Review*, 30:67–76.

McLeod, J. (2012) 'The meanings of stress', *Society and Mental Health*, 2: 172–186.

McLeod, J., Uemura, R. and Rohrman, S. (2012) 'Adolescent mental health, behavior problems, and academic achievement', *Journal of Health and Social Behavior*, 53(4): 482–497.

McMahon, R. (2020) 'The silenced manifesto: an autoethnography of living with Schizoaffective Disorder', PhD Dissertation, Wollongong: University of Wollongong.

McManus, S., Gunnell, D., Cooper, C., Bebbington, P., Howard, L., Brugha, T., Jenkins, R., Hassiotis, A., Weich, S. and Appleby, L. (2019) 'Prevalence of non-suicidal self-harm and service contact in England, 2000–14: repeated cross-sectional surveys of the general population', *The Lancet Psychiatry*, 6(7): 573–581.

McWade, B., Milton, D. and Beresford, P. (2015) 'Mad studies and neurodiversity: a dialogue', *Disability & Society*, 30:2: 305–309.

Mead, M. (1928) *Coming of Age in Samoa*, New York, NY: Morrow.

Mersky, J., Janczewski, C. and Nitkowski, J. (2018) 'Poor mental health among low-income women in the U.S.: The roles of adverse childhood and adult experiences', *Social Science and Medicine*, 206: 14–21.

Metzl, J. (2010) *Protest Psychosis: How Schizophrenia Became a Black Disease*, Boston, MA: Beacon Press.

Meurk, C., Carter, A., Partridge, B., Lucke, J. and Hall, W. (2014) 'How is acceptance of the brain disease model of addiction related to Australians' attitudes towards addicted individuals and treatments for addiction?', *BMC Psychiatry*, 14: 373–383.

Meyer, I. (2003) 'Prejudice, social stress, and mental health in lesbian, gay, and bisexual populations: conceptual issues and research evidence', *Psychological bulletin*, 129: 674–697.

Mezuk, B., Abdou, C., Hudson, D., Kershaw, K., Rafferty, J., Lee, H. and Jackson, J. (2013) '"White Box" epidemiology and the social neuroscience of health behaviors: The environmental affordances model', *Society and Mental Health*, 3(2): 79–95.

Miao, J., Wu, X. and Sun, X. (2019) 'Neighborhood, social cohesion, and the ELDERLY'S depression in Shanghai', *Social Science and Medicine*, 229: 134–143.

Migliore, S. (2001) 'From illness narratives to social commentary: A Pirandellian approach to "nerves"', *Medical Anthropology Quarterly*, 15: 100–125.

Miles, A. (1987 [1981]) *The Mentally Ill in Contemporary Society*, Oxford: Blackwell.

Miller, C., Solomon, S., Varni, S., Hodge, J., Knapp, A. and Bunn, J. (2016) 'A transactional approach to relationships over time between perceived HIV stigma and the psychological and physical well-being of people with HIV', *Social Science and* Medicine, 162: 97–105.

Mills, C. (2014) *Decolonizing Global Mental Health: The Psychiatrization of the Majority World*, London: Routledge.

Mills, C. (2018) '"Dead people don't claim": A psychopolitical autopsy of UK austerity suicides', *Critical Social Policy*, 38(2): 302–322.

Mills, C. and Klein, E. (2021) 'Affective technologies of welfare deterrence in Australia and the United Kingdom', *Economy and Society*, 50(3): 1–26.

Milner, A., Aitken, Z., Kavanagh, A., LaMontagne, A. and Petrie, D. (2017) 'Status inconsistency and mental health: A random effects and instrumental variables analysis using 14 annual waves of cohort data', *Social Science and Medicine*, 189: 129–137.

Mirdamadi, M. (2019) 'How does the death conscious culture of Iran affect experiences of depression?', *Culture, Medicine and Psychiatry*, 43(1):56–76.

Mirowsky, J. (1985) 'Depression and marital power: An equity model', *American Journal of Sociology*, 91: 557–592.

Mirowsky, J. (2007) 'The distribution's tail: A comment', *Health*, 11: 301–302.

Mirowsky, J. and Ross, C. (1983) 'Paranoia and the structure of powerlessness', *American Sociological Review*, 48(2): 228–239.

Mirowsky, J. and Ross, C. (1989) 'Psychiatric diagnosis as reified measurement', *Journal of Health and Social Behavior*, 30(1): 11–25.

Mishra, S. and Carleton, R. (2015) 'Subjective relative deprivation is associated with poorer physical and mental health', *Social Science and Medicine*, 147: 144–149.

Moncrieff, J. (2007) *The Myth of the Chemical Cure: A Critique of Psychiatric Drug Treatment*, Basingstoke: Palgrave.

Moncrieff, J. (2010) 'Psychiatric diagnosis as a political device', *Social Theory and Health*, 8: 370–382.

Montazer, S. and Wheaton, B. (2017) 'Economic conditions in countries of origin and trajectories in distress after migration to Canada: Results from the National Population Health Survey', *Society and Mental Health*, 7(1): 1–20.

Moran, G., Oz, G. and Karnieli-Miller, O. (2014) 'Psychiatrists' challenges in considering disclosure of schizophrenia diagnosis in Israel', *Qualitative Health Research*, 24(10): 1368–1380.

Mora-Rios, J., Ortega-Ortega, M. and Natera, G. (2016) 'Subjective experience and resources for coping with stigma in people with a diagnosis of schizophrenia: An intersectional approach', *Qualitative Health Research*, 26(5):697–711

Moreau, N. (2009) *État Dépressif et Temporalité: Contribution à la Sociologie de la Santé Mentale*, Montreal: Liber.

Moreno Pestaña, J.-L. (2006) 'Un cas de déviance dans les classes populaires: les seuils d'entrée dans les troubles alimentaires', *Cahiers d'Economie et de Sociologie Rurales*, 79: 67–95.

Morrall, P. (2000) *Madness and Murder*, London: Whurr.

Morrall, P. and Muir-Cochrane, E. (2002) 'Naked social control: Seclusion and psychiatric nursing in post-liberal society', *Australian e-Journal for the Advancement of Mental Health*, 1(2): 101–112.

Mort, M., Roberts, C. and Mackenzie, A. (2019) *Living Data: Making Sense of Health Bio-Sensing*, Bristol: Policy Press.

Moscone, F., Tosetti, E. and Vittadini, G. (2016) 'The impact of precarious employment on mental health: The case of Italy', *Social Science and Medicine*, 158: 86–95.

Moses, T. (2009) 'Self-labeling and its effects among adolescents diagnosed with mental disorders', *Social Science and Medicine*, 68: 570–578.

Moses, T. (2010) 'Being treated differently: Stigma experiences with family, peers, and school staff among adolescents with mental health disorders', *Social Science and* Medicine, 70: 985–993.

Moynihan, R., Gotzsche, P., Heath, I. and David, H. (2002) 'Selling sickness: The pharmaceutical industry and disease mongering', *BMJ*, 324(7342):886–891.

Mueller, A. and Abrutyn, S. (2016) 'Adolescents under pressure: A new Durkheimian framework for understanding adolescent suicide in a cohesive community', *American Sociological Review*, 81(5):877–99.

Muntaner, C., Eaton, W. and Diala, C. (2000) 'Social inequalities in mental health: A review of concepts and underlying assumptions', *Health*, 4(1): 89–113.

Muntaner, C., Ng, E., Vanroelen, C., Christ, S. and Eaton, W. (2013) 'Social stratification, social closure, and social class as determinants of mental health disparities', in C. Aneshensel, J. Phelan and A. Bierman (eds) *Handbook of the Sociology of Mental Health*, New York, NY: Springer, pp 205–227.

Murat, L. (2014) *The Man Who Thought He Was Napoleon: Toward a Political History of Madness*, Chicago, IL: University of Chicago Press.

Murphy, D. (2001) 'Hacking's reconciliation: Putting the biological and sociological together in the explanation of mental illness', *Philosophy of the Social Sciences*, 31(2): 139–162.

Murray, S. (2008) *Representing Autism: Culture, Narrative, Fascination*, Liverpool: Liverpool University Press.

Myers, N. (2010) 'Culture, stress and recovery from schizophrenia: Lessons from the field for global mental health', *Culture, Medicine, and Psychiatry*, 34(3): 500–528.

Nadesan, M. (2005) *Constructing Autism: Unravelling the 'Truth' and Understanding the Social*, London: Routledge.

Nakamura, K. (2013) *A Disability of The Soul: an Ethnography of Schizophrenia and Mental Illness in Contemporary Japan*, New York, NY: Cornell University Press.

Nazroo, J., Bhui, K. and Rhodes, J. (2020) 'Where next for understanding race/ethnic inequalities in severe mental illness? Structural, interpersonal and institutional racism', *Sociology of Health and Illness*, 42(2): 262–276.

Nelson, A. (2019) 'Diagnostic dissonance and negotiations of biomedicalisation: Mental health practitioners' resistance to the DSM technology and diagnostic standardisation', *Sociology of Health and Illness*, 41(5): 933–949.

Neria, Y., Gross, R. and Marshall, R. (eds) (2006) *9/11: Mental Health in the Wake of Terrorist Attacks*, Cambridge: Cambridge University Press.

Nettleton, S., Burrows, R. and O'Malley, L. (2005) 'The mundane realities of the everyday lay use of the internet for health, and their consequences for media convergence', *Sociology of Health and Illness*, 27(7): 972–992.

Newman, C., Smith, A., Duck-Chong, E., Vivienne, S., Davies, C., Robinson, K. and Aggleton, P. (2021) 'Waiting to be seen: Social perspectives on trans health', *Health Sociology Review*, 30(1): 1–8.

Ng, E. (2009) 'Heartache of the state, enemy of the self: Bipolar disorder and cultural change in urban China', *Cult Med Psychiatry*, 33(3): 421–450.

Ng, E. (2020) *A Time of Lost Gods: Mediumship, Madness, and the Ghost after Mao*, Oakland, CA: University of California Press.

NIC (National Intelligence Council) (2021) *Global Trends 2040*, Available from: https://www.dni.gov/index.php/gt2040-home [Accessed 3 February 2022]

Niehaus, I. (2012) 'Gendered endings: Narratives of male and female suicides in the South African Lowveld', *Culture, Medicine, and Psychiatry*, 36(2): 327–347.

Nielsen, L., Koushede, V., Vinther-Larsen, M., Bendtsen, P., Kjær Ersbøll, A., Due, P. and Holstein, B. (2015) 'Does school social capital modify socioeconomic inequality in mental health? A multi-level analysis in Danish schools', *Social Science and Medicine*, 140: 35–43.

Nishimura, J. (2011) 'Socioeconomic status and depression across Japan, Korea, and China: Exploring the impact of labor market structures', *Social Science and Medicine*, 73(4): 604–614.

Noh, S. and Avison, W. (1996) 'Asian immigrants and the stress process: A study of Koreans in Canada', *Journal of Health and Social Behavior*, 37(2): 192–206.

Nowotny, K., Peterson, R. and Boardman, J. (2015) 'Gendered contexts: Variation in suicidal ideation by female and male youth across U.S. states', *Journal of Health and Social Behavior*, 56(1): 114–130.

O'Donnell, A., Stuart, J. and O'Donnell, K. (2020) 'The long-term financial and psychological resettlement outcomes of pre-migration trauma and post-settlement difficulties in resettled refugees', *Social Science and Medicine*, 262: 113246.

OECD (2018) *Health at a Glance*, Brussels: OECD

Olcoń, K. and Gulbas, L. (2018) '"Because that's the culture": Providers' perspectives on the mental health of Latino immigrant youth', *Qualitative Health Research*, 28(12): 1944–1954.

Oliffe, J., Broom, A., Popa, M., Jenkins, E., Rice, S., Ferlatte, O. and Rossnagel, E. (2019) 'Unpacking social isolation in men's suicidality', *Qualitative Health Research*, 29(3): 315–327.

O'Reilly, M., Muskett, T., Karim, K. and Lester, J. (2020) 'Parents' constructions of normality and pathology in child mental health assessments', *Sociology of Health and Illness*, 42(3): 544–564.

Orr, J. (2006) *Panic Diaries: A Genealogy of Panic Disorder*, Durham, NC: Duke University Press.

Ortega, F. (2009) 'The cerebral subject and the challenge of neurodiversity', *BioSocieties*, 4(4): 425–445.

Owens, J. (2020) 'Social class, diagnoses of attention-deficit/hyperactivity disorder, and child well-being', *Journal of Health and Social Behavior*, 61(2): 134–152.

Parsons, T. (1951) *The Social System*, Glencoe, IL: The Free Press.

Patel, V. and Winston, M. (1994) '"Universality of mental illness" revisited: Assumptions, artefacts and new directions', *British Journal of Psychiatry*, 165(4): 437–440.

Pathare, S., Brazinova, A. and Levav, I. (2018) 'Care gap: A comprehensive measure to quantify unmet needs in mental health', *Epidemiology and Psychiatric Sciences*, 27(5): 463–46.

Payton, A. and Thoits, P. (2011) 'Medicalization, Direct-to-Consumer Advertising, and Mental Illness Stigma', *Society and Mental Health*, 1(1): 55–70.

Pearlin, L. (1989) 'The sociological study of stress', *Journal of Health and Social Behavior*, 30(3): 241–256.

Pearlin, L., Menaghan, E., Lieberman, M. and Mullan, J. (1981) 'The stress process', *Journal of Health and Social Behavior*, 22(4), 337–356.

Pearson, V. and Liu, M. (2002) 'Ling's death: An ethnography of a Chinese woman's suicide', *Suicide and Life-Threatening Behavior*, 32(4): 347–358.

Perales, F. and Todd, A. (2018) 'Structural stigma and the health and wellbeing of Australian LGB populations: Exploiting geographic variation in the results of the 2017 same-sex marriage plebiscite', *Social Science and Medicine*, 208: 190–199.

Perry, A., Lawrence, V. and Henderson, C. (2020) 'Stigmatisation of those with mental health conditions in the acute general hospital setting. A qualitative framework synthesis', *Social Science and* Medicine, 255: 112974.

Perry, B. (2011) 'The labeling paradox: Stigma, the sick role, and social networks in mental illness', *Journal of Health and Social Behavior*, 52(4): 460–477.

Pescosolido, B. (2013) 'The public stigma of mental illness: What do we think; what do we know; what can we prove?', *Journal of Health and Social Behavior*, 54(1): 1–21.

Pescosolido, B., Manago, B. and Monahan, J. (2019) 'Evolving public views on the likelihood of violence from people with mental illness: Stigma and its consequences', *Health Affairs*, 38(10): 1735–1743.

Pescosolido, B., Martin, J., Lang, S. and Ólafsdóttir, S. (2008) 'Rethinking theoretical approaches to stigma: A Framework Integrating Normative Influences on Stigma (FINIS)', *Social Science & Medicine*, 67(3): 431–440.

Phelan, J. (2005) 'Geneticization of deviant behavior and consequences for stigma: The case of mental illness', *Journal of Health and Social Behavior*, 46(4): 307–322.

Phillips, J. (2014) 'A changing epidemiology of suicide? The influence of birth cohorts on suicide rates in the United States', *Social Science and Medicine*, 114: 151–160.

Pickersgill, M. (2011) '"Promising" therapies: Neuroscience, clinical practice, and the treatment of psychopathy', *Sociology of Health & Illness*, 33(3), 448–464.

Pickersgill, M. (2020) 'Uncertainty work as ontological negotiation: Adjudicating access to therapy in clinical psychology', *Sociolology of Health Illness*, 42(1): 84–98.

Pickersgill, M., Niewöhner, J., Müller, R., Martin, P. and Cunningham-Burley, S. (2013) 'Mapping the new molecular landscape: Social dimensions of epigenetics', *New Genetics and Society*, 32(4): 429–447.

Picone, M. (2012) 'Suicide and the afterlife: Popular religion and the standardisation of "culture" in Japan', *Culture, Medicine, and Psychiatry*, 36(2): 391–408.

Piercy, M. (1976) *Woman on the Edge of Time*, New York, NY: Knopf.

Pietila, I. and Rytkonen, M. (2008) 'Coping with stress and by stress: Russian men and women talking about transition, stress and health', *Social Science and Medicine*, 66(2): 327–338.

Pike, K. and Borovoy, A. (2004) 'The rise of eating disorders in Japan: Issues of culture and limitations of the model of "westernization"', *Culture, Medicine, and Psychiatry*, 28(4): 493–531.

Piketty, T. (2017) *Capital in the Twenty-First Century*, Cambridge, MA: Harvard University Press.

Pilgrim, D. (2007) 'The survival of psychiatric diagnosis', *Social Science and Medicine*, 65(3):536–47.

Pilgrim, D. and Rogers, A. (2002) *Mental Health and Inequality*, London: Red Globe Press.

Pilgrim, D. and Rogers, A. (2005) 'The troubled relationship between psychiatry and sociology', *International Journal of Social Psychiatry*, 51(3), 228–241.

Pinto, S. (2014) *Daughters of Parvati: Women and Madness in Contemporary India*, Philadelphia, PA: University of Pennsylvania Press.

Pirkis, J., Ftanou, M., Williamson, M., Machlin, A., Spittal, M., Bassilios, B. and Harris, M. (2011) 'Australia's Better Access initiative: an evaluation', *Australia and New Zealand Journal of Psychiatry*, 45(9):726–739.

Pitts, J. (1968) 'Social control: The concept' in D. Sills (ed) *International Encyclopedia of Social Sciences*, New York, NY: Macmillan, pp 381–396.

Platt, J., Bates, L., Jager, J., McLaughlin, K. and Keyes, K. (2020) 'Changes in the depression gender gap from 1992 to 2014: Cohort effects and mediation by gendered social position', *Social Science and Medicine*, 258: 113088.

Pollner, M. (1978) 'Constitutive and mundane versions of labeling theory', *Human Studies*, 1(1): 269–288.

Pols, H. (2018) *Nurturing Indonesia: Medicine and Decolonisation in the Dutch East Indies*, Cambridge: Cambridge University Press.

Pope, L. (2015) 'To forgive and discredit: Bipolar identities and medicated selves among female youth in residential treatment', *Culture, Medicine, and Psychiatry*, 39(3): 505–531.

Price-Robertson, R., Manderson, L. and Duff, C. (2017) 'Mental ill health, recovery and the family assemblage', *Culture, Medicine, and Psychiatry*, 41(3): 407–430.

Prickett, P. (2021) 'When the road is covered in nails: Making sense of madness in an urban mosque', *Social Problems*, 68(1): 136–151.

Pringle, Y. (2019) *Psychiatry and Decolonisation in Uganda*, London: Palgrave.

Prins, S., Bates, L., Keyes, K. and Muntaner, C. (2015) 'Anxious? Depressed? You might be suffering from capitalism: Contradictory class locations and the prevalence of depression and anxiety in the USA', *Sociology of Health and Illness*, 37(8): 1352–1372.

Prior, P. (1999) *Gender and Mental Health*, London: Macmillan.

Prior, S. (2012) 'Overcoming stigma: How young people position themselves as counselling service users', *Sociology of Health and Illness*, 34(5): 697–713.

Pryor, L., Strandberg-Larsen, K., Nybo-Andersen, A-M., Hulvej-Rod, N. and Melchior, M. (2019) 'Trajectories of family poverty and children's mental health: Results from the Danish National Birth Cohort', *Social Science and Medicine*, 220: 371–378.

REFERENCES

Qi, D. and Wu, Y. (2018) 'Does welfare stigma exist in China? Policy evaluation of the Minimum Living Security System on recipients' psychological health and wellbeing', *Social Science and Medicine*, 205: 26–36.

Quinn, D., Weisz, B. and Lawner, E. (2017) 'Impact of active concealment of stigmatized identities on physical and psychological quality of life', *Social Science and Medicine*, 192: 14–17.

Quintaneiro, T. (2006) 'The concept of figuration or configuration in Norbert Elias' sociological theory', *Teoria & Sociedade*, 2: Online.

Rafalovich, A. (2005) 'Exploring clinician uncertainty in the diagnosis and treatment of attention deficit hyperactivity disorder', *Sociology of Health and Illness*, 27(3): 305–23.

Rahimi, S. (2015) *Meaning, Madness and Political Subjectivity: A Study of Schizophrenia and Culture in Turkey*, London: Routledge.

Rapp, R. (2011) 'A child surrounds this brain: The future of neurological difference according to scientists, parents and diagnosed young adults', in M. Pickersgill and I. Van Neulen (eds) *Sociological Reflections on the Neurosciences*, Bingley: Emerald, pp 3–26.

Reay, B., Attwood, N., and Gooder, C. (2015) *Sex Addiction: A Critical History*, Cambridge: Polity Press.

Rees, S. and Silove, D. (2011) 'Sakit Hati: A state of chronic mental distress related to resentment and anger amongst West Papuan refugees exposed to persecution', *Social Science and Medicine*, 73(1): 103–10.

Reiss, F. (2013) 'Socioeconomic inequalities and mental health problems in children and adolescents: A systematic review', *Social Science and Medicine*, 90: 24–31.

Reith, G. (2013) 'Techno economic systems and excessive consumption', *The British Journal of Sociology*, 64(4): 717–738.

Rens, E., Dom, G., Remmen, R., Michielsen, J. and Van den Broech, K. (2020) 'Unmet mental health needs in the general population: Perspectives of Belgian health and social care professionals' *International Journal of Equity Health*, 19(1): 169–179.

Reyes-García, V., Gravlee, C., McDade, T., Huanca, T., Leonard, W. and Tanner, S. (2010) 'Cultural consonance and psychological well-being. Estimates using longitudinal data from an Amazonian society', *Culture, Medicine, and Psychiatry*, 34(1):186–203.

Reynolds, K., Medved, M., Mackenzie, C., Funk, L. and Koven, L. (2020) 'Older adults' narratives of seeking mental health treatment: Making sense of mental health challenges and "muddling through" to care', *Qualitative Health Research*, 30(10): 1517–1528.

Rice, N., Grealy, M., Javaid, A. and Serrano, R.M. (2011) 'Understanding the social interaction difficulties of women with unipolar depression', *Qualitative Health Research*, 21(10): 1388–1399.

Richards, D. (1996) 'Strangers in a strangle land: Expatriate paranoia and the dynamics of exclusion', *The International Journal of Human Resource Management*, 7(2): 553–571.

Ridge, D., Emslie, C. and White, A. (2011) 'Understanding how men experience, express and cope with mental distress: Where next?', *Sociology of Health and Illness*, 33(1): 145–159.

Riumallo-Herl, C., Kawachi, I. and Avendano, M. (2014) 'Social capital, mental health and biomarkers in Chile: Assessing the effects of social capital in a middle-income country', *Social Science and Medicine*, 105: 47–58.

River, J. and Flood, M. (2021) 'Masculinities, emotions and men's suicide', *Sociology of Heath and Illness*, 43(4): 910–927.

Roberts, C. and McWade, B. (2021) 'Messengers of stress: Towards a cortisol sociology', *Sociology of Health & Illness*, 43(4): 895–909.

Roberts, R. (2015) *Psychology & Capitalism*, Winchester: Zero Books.

Rockett, I., Samora, J. and Cohen, J. (2006) 'The black-white suicide paradox: possible effects of misclassification', *Social Science and Medicine*, 63(8): 2165–2175.

Rogers, A. and Pilgrim, D. (2014) *A Sociology of Mental Health and Illness*, Milton Keynes: Open University Press.

Romero, M.C., Ruiz, A.L. and Melluish, S. (2020) 'Reimagining "mental health" from the cosmovision of *Abya Yala* (Latin America)', *International Review of Psychiatry*, 32(4): 299–302.

Rose, D. (2020) 'On personal epiphanies and collective knowledge in survivor research and action', *Social Theory and Health*, 18(2): 110–122.

Rosa, H. (2015) *Social Acceleration: A New Theory of Modernity*, New York, NY: Columbia University Press.

Rose, N. (1988) 'Calculable minds and manageable individuals', *History of the Human Sciences*, 1(2): 179–200.

Rose, N. (1990) *Governing the Soul: The Shaping of the Private Self*, London: Routledge.

Rose, N. (1996) *Inventing our Selves: Psychology, Power, and Personhood*, Cambridge: Cambridge University Press.

Rose, N. (2007) *The Politics of Life Itself: Biomedicine, Power, and Subjectivity in the Twenty-First Century*, Princeton, NJ: Princeton University Press.

Rose, N. (2018) *Our Psychiatric Futures*. Cambridge: Polity Press.

Rosenfield, S. (2012) 'Triple jeopardy? Mental health at the intersection of gender, race, and class', *Social Science and Medicine*, 74(11): 1791–1801.

Rosenfield, S. and Mouzon, D. (2013) 'Gender and mental health' in C.S. Aneshensel, J.C. Phelan and A. Bierman (eds) *Handbook of the Sociology of Mental Health*, Dordrecht: Springer, pp 277–296.

Rosenhan, D. (1973) 'On being sane in insane places', *Science*, 179(4070): 250–258.

Ross Arguedas, A. (2020) '"Can naughty be healthy?": Healthism and its discontents in news coverage of orthorexia nervosa', *Social Science and Medicine*, 246: 112784.

Ross, C., Reynolds, J. and Geis, K. (2000) 'The contingent meaning of neighborhood stability for residents' psychological well-being', *American Sociological Review*, 65(4): 581–597.

Rowe, P. and Guerin, B. (2018) 'Contextualizing the mental health of metal youth: A community for social protection, identity, and musical empowerment', *Journal of Community Psychology*, 47(4): 429–441.

Roy, M., Rivest, M.P., Namian, D. and Moreau, N. (2019) 'The critical reception of the DSM-5: Towards a typology of audiences', *Public Understanding of Science*, 28(8): 932–948.

Ruiz, M., Malyutina, S., Pajak, A., Kozela, M., Kubinova, R. and Bobak, M. (2019) 'Congruent relations between perceived neighbourhood social cohesion and depressive symptoms among older European adults: An East-West analysis', *Social Science and Medicine*, 237: 112454.

Ruiz-Junco, N. and Brossard, B. (2018) *Updating Charles H. Cooley: Contemporary Perspectives on a Sociological Classic*, London: Routledge.

Russell, F. (2018) 'Wages for self-care: Mental illness and reproductive labour', *Cultural Studies Review*, 24(2): 26–38.

Ruth, R. and Santacruz, E. (eds) (2017) *LGBT Psychology and Mental Health: Emerging Research and Advances*, Santa Barbara, CA: Praeger.

Sadler, J. (2004) *Values and Psychiatric Diagnosis*, Oxford: Oxford University Press.

Sadler, M., Meagor, E. and Kaye, K. (2012) 'Stereotypes of mental disorders differ in competence and warmth', *Social Science and Medicine*, 74(6): 915–922.

Sakurai, K., Kawakami, N., Yamaoka, N., Ishikawa, H. and Hashimoto, H. (2010) 'The impact of subjective and objective social status on psychological distress among men and women in Japan', *Social Science and Medicine*, 70(11): 1832–1839.

Sartorius, N. (2007) 'Stigma and mental health', *The Lancet*, 370(9590): 810–811.

Satariano, B. (2019) 'Diverse socioeconomic processes influencing health and wellbeing across generations in deprived neighbourhoods in Malta', *Social Science and Medicine*, 232: 453–459.

Sato, K., Kuroda, S. and Owan, H. (2020) 'Mental health effects of long work hours, night and weekend work, and short rest periods', *Social Science and Medicine*, 246: 112774.

Sayad, A. (2004) *The Suffering of the Immigrant*, Cambridge: Polity Press.

Scambler, G. (2018) 'Heaping blame on shame: "Weaponising stigma" for neoliberal times', *The Sociological Review*, 66(4); 766–782.

Scheff, T. (1966) *Being Mentally Ill. A Sociological Theory*, Chicago, IL: Aldine de Gruyter.

Scheff, T. (1974) 'The labelling theory of mental illness', *American Sociological Review*, 39(3): 444–452.

Scheff, T. (1975) 'Reply to Chauncey and Gove', *American Sociological Review*, 40(2): 252–256.

Scheper-Hughes, N. (1977) *Saints, Scholars and Schizophrenics: Mental Illness in Rural Ireland*, Berkeley, CA: University of California Press.

Schieman, S. (2019) 'Ordinary lives and the sociological character of stress: How work, family, and status contribute to emotional inequality', *Society and Mental Health*, 9(2): 127–142.

Schieman, S. and Plickert, G. (2007) 'Functional limitations and changes in levels of depression among older adults: A multiple-hierarchy stratification perspective', *The Journals of Gerontology*, 62(1): S36–S4.

Schieman, S., Kurashina, Y. and Van Gundy, K. (2006) 'The nature of work and the stress of higher status', *Journal of Health and Social Behavior*, 47(3): 242–257.

Schmitz, R., Robinson, B.A., Tabler, J., Welch, B. and Rafaquit, S. (2019) 'LGBTQ+ Latino/a young people's interpretations of stigma and mental health: An intersectional minority stress perspective', *Society and Mental Health*, 10(2): 163–179.

Schnittker, J. (2010) 'Gene-environment correlations in the stress-depression relationship', *Journal of Health and Social Behavior*, 51(3): 229–243.

Schnittker, J. (2020) *The Diagnostic System: Why the Classification of Psychiatric Disorders Is Necessary, Difficult, and Never Settled*, New York, NY: Columbia University Press.

Schoon, I. and Bynner, J. (2003) 'Risk and resilience in the life course: Implications for interventions and social policies', *Journal of Youth Studies* (6)1: 21–31.

Schulze, B. and Angermeyer, M.C. (2003) 'Subjective experiences of stigma. A focus group study of schizophrenic patients, their relatives and mental health professionals', *Social Science and Medicine*, 56(2): 299–312.

Schwartz, O. (2011) 'La pénétration de la "culture psychologique de masse" dans un groupe populaire: paroles de conducteurs de bus', *Sociologie*, 2(4): 345–361.

Schwartz, S. (2002) 'Outcomes for the sociology of mental health: Are we meeting our goals?', *Journal of Health and Social Behavior*, 43(2): 223–235.

Schwartz, S. (2007) 'Distinguishing distress from disorder as psychological outcomes of stressful social arrangements: Can we and should we?', *Health*, 11(3): 291–299.

Schwartz, S. and Meyer, I. (2010) 'Mental health disparities research: The impact of within and between group analyses on tests of social stress hypotheses', *Social Science and Medicine*, 70: 1111–1118.

Schweingruber, D. and Wahl, D. (2019) 'Whither the internal conversation?', *Symbolic Interaction*, 42(3): 351–373.

Scott, S. (2006) 'The medicalisation of shyness: From social misfits to social fitness', *Sociology of Health and Illness*, 28(2): 133–53.

Scott, S., Munoz, E., Mogle, J., Gamaldo, A., Smyth, J., Almeida, D. and Sliwinski, M. (2018) 'Perceived neighborhood characteristics predict severity and emotional response to daily stressors', *Social Science and Medicine*, 200: 262–270.

Scott, W. (1990) 'PTSD in DSM-III: A case in the politics of diagnosis and disease', *Social Problems*, 37(3): 294–310.

Scull, A. (1989) *Social Order / Mental Disorder*, Berkeley, CA: University of California Press.

Scull, A. (2019) *Psychiatry and Its Discontents*, Oakland, CA: University of California Press.

Seligman, R. and Kirmayer, L. (2008) 'Dissociative experience and cultural neuroscience: Narrative, metaphor and mechanism', *Culture, Medicine, and Psychiatry*, 32(1): 31–64.

Selye, H. (1956) *The Stress of Life*, London: McGraw-Hill.

Seng, J., Lopez, W., Sperlich, M., Hamama, L. and Reed Meldrum, C. (2012) 'Marginalized identities, discrimination burden, and mental health: Empirical exploration of an interpersonal-level approach to modeling intersectionality', *Social Science and Medicine*, 75(12): 2437–45.

Sepúlveda Jara, R. and Oyarce Pisani, A.M. (2020) 'New and old knowledge aimed at decolonising mental health: Reflections and proposals from Chile', *International Review of Psychiatry*, 32(4): 334–339.

Sercu, C. and Bracke, P. (2017) 'Stigma, social structure, and the biomedical framework: Exploring the stigma experiences of inpatient service users in two Belgian psychiatric hospitals', *Qualitative Health Research*, 27(8): 1249–1261.

Shellae Versey, H., Cogburn, C., Wilkins, C. and Joseph, N. (2019) 'Appropriated racial oppression: Implications for mental health in Whites and Blacks', *Social Science and Medicine*, 230: 295–302.

Sherlock, S. and Kielich, L. (1991) 'Medication and the patient role: Implications for the labeling theory of mental illness', *Michigan Sociological Review*, 5: 90–102.

Sherman, A., Clark, K., Robinson, K., Noorani, T. and Poteat, T. (2020) 'Trans* community connection, health, and wellbeing: A systematic review', *LGBT Health*, 7(1): 1–14.

Sherman, R. (2017) *Uneasy Street: The Anxieties of Affluence*, Princeton, NJ: Princeton University Press.

Shildrick, T. (2018) 'Lessons from Grenfell: Poverty propaganda, stigma and class power', *The Sociological Review*, 66(4): 783–798.

Shorer, S., Goldblatt, H., Caspi, Y. and Azaiza, F. (2018) 'Culture as a double-edged sword: The posttraumatic experience of indigenous ethnic minority veterans', *Qualitative Health Research*, 28(5): 766–777.

Shorter, E. (2013) *How Everyone Became Depressed: The Rise and Fall of the Nervous Breakdown*, Oxford: Oxford University Press.

Simbayi, L., Kalichman, S., Strebel, A., Cloete, A., Henda, N. and Mqeketoet, A. (2007) 'Internalized stigma, discrimination, and depression among men and women living with HIV/AIDS in Cape Town, South Africa', *Social Science and Medicine*, 64(9): 1823–1831.

Simmel, G. (2010) 'The metropolis and mental life' in G. Bridge and S. Watson (eds) *The Blackwell City Reader*, Oxford: Blackwell, pp 103–111.

Simon, R. (2002) 'Revisiting the relationships among gender, marital status, and mental health', *American Journal of Sociology*, 107(4): 1065–1096.

Simon, R. (2020) 'Gender, emotions, and mental health in the United States: Patterns, explanations, and new directions', *Society and Mental Health*, 10(2): 97–111.

Singh, I. (2011) 'A disorder of anger and aggression: Children's perspectives on attention deficit/hyperactivity disorder in the UK', *Social Science and Medicine*, 73(6): 889–896.

Skovbo Rasmussen, P., Kryger Pedersen, I. and Pagsberg. A.K. (2020) 'Biographical disruption or cohesion?: How parents deal with their child's autism diagnosis', *Social Science & Medicine*, 244, 112673.

Smardon, R. (2008) '"I'd rather not take Prozac": stigma and commodification in antidepressant consumer narratives', *Health*, 12(1): 67–86.

Snedker, K.A. (2016) 'Unburdening stigma: Identity repair through rituals in mental health court', *Society and Mental Health*, 6(1): 36–55.

Song, J., Mailick, M. and Greenberg, J. (2018) 'Health of parents of individuals with developmental disorders or mental health problems: Impacts of stigma', *Social Science and Medicine*, 217: 152–158.

Song, L. (2011) 'Social capital and psychological distress', *Journal of Health and Social Behavior*, 52(4): 478–492.

Souza Prado, G.A. (2020) 'Coloniality and perspectivism in psychology: From damnation to ecosophical care relations', *International Review of Psychiatry*, 32(4): 320–326.

Speed, E., Moncrieff, J. and Rapley, M. (eds) (2014) *De-Medicalizing Misery II: Society, Politics and the Mental Health Industry*, London: Palgrave.

Spoont, M., Sayer, N., Friedemann-Sanchez, G., Parker, L., Murdoch, M. and Chiros, C. (2009) 'From trauma to PTSD: beliefs about sensations, symptoms, and mental illness', *Qualitative Health Research*, 19(10): 1456–1465.

REFERENCES

Srole, L., Langner, T., Michael, S., Opler, M. and Rennie, T. (1962) *Mental Health in the Metropolis: The Midtown Manhattan Study*, New York, NY: McGraw-Hill.

St Guillaume, L. and Finlay, E. (2018) 'Disabled mobility and the production of impairment: The case of Australia's migration policy framework', *Asia and Pacific Viewpoint*, 59: 119–131.

Stack, S. (2000) 'Suicide: A 15-year review of the sociological literature. Part I: Cultural and economic factors', *Suicide and Life Threatening Behavior*, 30: 145–162.

Staub, M. (2011) *Madness is Civilization: When the Diagnosis was Social, 1948–1980*, Chicago, IL: University of Chicago Press.

Steggals, P. (2015) *Making Sense of Self-Harm*, London: Palgrave.

Steggals, P., Lawler, S. and Graham, R. (2020) 'The social life of self-injury: exploring the communicative dimension of a very personal practice', *Sociology of Health & Illness*, 42: 157–170.

Stephen, M. and Suryani, K. (2000) 'Shamanism, psychosis and autonomous imagination', *Culture, Medicine, and Psychiatry*, 24: 5–38.

Stockdale, S., Wells, K., Tanga, L., Belinc, T., Zhanga, L. and Sherbourne, C. (2007) 'The importance of social context: Neighborhood stressors, stress-buffering mechanisms, and alcohol, drug, and mental health disorders', *Social Science and Medicine*, 65(9): 1867–1881.

Stocking, G. (ed) (1991) *Colonial Situations: Essays on the Contextualization of Ethnographic Knowledge*, Madison, WI: Univ. of Wisconsin Press.

Sullivan, O., Gershuny, J. and Robinson, J. (2018) 'Stalled or uneven gender revolution? A long-term processual framework for understanding why change is slow', *Journal of Family Theory & Review*, 10(2): 263–279.

Sulzer, S. (2015) 'Does "difficult patient" status contribute to de facto demedicalization? The case of borderline personality disorder', *Social Science and Medicine*, 142: 82–89.

Summerfield, D. (2000) 'Conflict and health: War and mental health: A brief overview', *BMJ*, 321: 232–236.

Summerfield, D. (2012) 'Afterword: Against "global mental health"', *Transcultural Psychiatry*, 49(3–4): 519–530.

Summerfield, D. (2013) '"Global mental health" is an oxymoron and medical imperialism', *BMJ*, 346: f3509.

Sun, A. and Houle, J. (2018) 'Trajectories of unsecured debt across the life course and mental health at midlife', *Society and Mental Health*, 10(1): 61–79.

Swanton, T. and Gainsbury, S. (2020) 'Debt stress partly explains the relationship between problem gambling and comorbid mental health problems', *Social Science and Medicine*, 265: 113476.

Sweet, E. (2018) '"Like you failed at life": Debt, health and neoliberal subjectivity', *Social Science and Medicine*, 212: 86–93.

Taguibao, C. and Rosenheck, R. (2021) 'Medical education and the stigmatization of mental illness in the Philippines', *Culture, Medicine, and Psychiatry*, 45: 312–331.

Takeuchi, D. (2016) 'Vintage wine in new bottles: Infusing select ideas into the study of immigration, immigrants, and mental health', *Journal of Health and Social Behavior*, 57(4): 423–435.

Takeuchi, D. and Gage, S.-Y. (2003) 'What to do with race? Changing notions of race in the social sciences', *Culture, Medicine and Psychiatry*, 27: 435–445.

Takeuchi, D. and Williams, D. (2003) 'Race, ethnicity and mental health: Introduction to the Special Issue', *Journal of Health and Social Behavior*, 44(3): 233–236.

Tan, C. (2018) '"I'm a normal autistic person, not an abnormal neurotypical": Autism Spectrum Disorder diagnosis as biographical illumination', *Social Science and Medicine*, 197:161–167.

Taylor, C. (2016) '"Relational by nature"? Men and women do not differ in physiological response to social stressors faced by token women', *American Journal of Sociology*, 122(1): 49–89.

Taylor, K. (2019) 'Pornography addiction: The fabrication of a transient sexual disease', *History of Human Sciences*, 32(5): 56–83.

Tekin, S. (2014) 'The missing self in Hacking's looping effects' in H. Kincaid and J.A. Sullivan (eds) *Classifying Psychopathology: Mental Kinds and Natural Kinds*, Cambridge, MA: MIT Press, pp 1–10.

Townsend, P., Davidson, N., Black, D., and Whitehead, M. (1988) *Inequalities in Health: The Black Report*, London: Penguin.

Thoits, P. (1985) 'Self-labeling processes in mental illness: The role of emotional deviance', *The American Journal of Sociology*, 91(2): 221–249.

Thoits, P. (1995) 'Stress, coping, and social support processes: Where are we? What next?', *Journal of Health and Social Behavior*, S: 53–79.

Thoits, P.A. (2010) 'Stress and health: Major findings and policy implications', *Journal of Health and Social Behavior*, 51: 41–53.

Thoits, P. (2013) 'Self, identity, stress, and mental health' in C. Aneshensel, J. Phelan and A. Bierman (eds) *Handbook of the Sociology of Mental Health*, second edition, Dordrecht: Springer, pp 357–377.

Thoits, P. (2017) 'Sociological approaches to mental illness' in E. Wright and T. Scheid (eds) *A Handbook for the Study of Mental Health: Social Contexts, Theories, and Systems*, Cambridge: Cambridge University Press, pp 126–144.

Thoits, P. and Link, B. (2016) 'Stigma resistance and well-being among people in treatment for psychosis', *Society and Mental Health*, 6(1): 1–20.

Thomas, F., Wyatt, K. and Hansford, L. (2020) 'The violence of narrative: Embodying responsibility for poverty-related stress', *Sociology of Health and Illness*, 42(5): 1123–1138.

Tiffin, P., Pearce, M. and Parker, L. (2005) 'Social mobility over the lifecourse and self-reported mental health at age 50: Prospective cohort study', *Journal of Epidemiology and Community Health*, 59(10): 870–872.

Timmermans, S. and Tietbohl, C. (2018) 'Fifty years of sociological leadership at Social Science and Medicine', *Social Science & Medicine*, 196: 209–215.

Townsend, P., Davidson, N., Black, D. and Whitehead, M. (1988) *Inequalities in Health: The Black Report*, London: Penguin.

Tran, A. (2017) 'Neurasthenia, generalized anxiety disorder, and the medicalization of worry in a Vietnamese psychiatric hospital', *Medical Anthropology Quarterly*, 31(2): 198–217.

Tseris, E. (2019) *Trauma, Women's Mental Health, and Social Justice: Pitfalls and Possibilities*, Abingdon: Routledge.

Tsou, J. (2007) 'Hacking on the looping effects of psychiatric classifications: What is an interactive and indifferent kind?', *International Studies in the Philosophy of Sciences*, 21(3): 329–344.

Tsou, J. (2016) 'Natural kinds, psychiatric classification and the history of the DSM', *History of Psychiatry*, 27(4): 406–424.

Tudor, A. (2017) 'Dimensions of transnationalism', *Feminist Review*, 117(1): 20–40.

Tudor, A. (2019) 'Im/possibilities of refusing and choosing gender', *Feminist Theory*, 20(4): 361–380.

Turcios, C. (2017) 'Questioning the paradox: How Mexican and Central America's Northern Triangle immigrants describe the difficulties of immigration and life in the United States', MA Dissertation, College Park, MD: University of Maryland.

Turner, B. and Luna Sánchez, S.E. (2020) 'The legacy of colonialism in Guatemala and its impact on the psychological and mental health of indigenous Mayan communities', *International Review of Psychiatry*, 32(4): 313–319.

Turner, R. (2013) 'Understanding health disparities', *Society and Mental Health*, 3(3): 170–186.

Turner, R., Russell, D., Glover, R. and Hutto, P. (2007) 'The social antecedents of anger proneness in young adulthood', *Journal of Health and Social Behavior*, 48(1): 68–83.

Tyler, I. (2018) 'Resituating Erving Goffman: From stigma power to Black power', *The Sociological Review*, 66(4): 744–765.

Tyler, I. (2020) *Stigma: The Machinery of Inequality*, London: Zed Books.

Tyler, I. and Slater, T. (2018) 'Rethinking the sociology of stigma', *The Sociological Review*, 66(4): 721–743.

Tzeng, W.-C. and Lipson, J.G. (2004) 'The cultural context of suicide stigma in Taiwan', *Qualitative Health Research*, 14(3): 345–358.

Ussher, J. (2011) *The Madness of Women: Myth and Experience*, Hove: Routledge.

Valdez, C., Chavez, T. and Woulfe, J. (2013) 'Emerging adults' lived experience of formative family stress: The family's lasting influence', *Qualitative Health Research*, 23(8): 1089–1102.

Valentine, K. (2010) 'A consideration of medicalisation: Choice, engagement and other responsibilities of parents of children with autism spectrum disorder', *Social Science and Medicine*, 71(5): 950–957.

Vallee, J., Cadot, E., Roustit, C., Parizot, I. and Chauvin, P. (2011) 'The role of daily mobility in mental health inequalities: The interactive influence of activity space and neighbourhood of residence on depression', *Social Science and Medicine*, 73(8): 1133–1144.

Van de Velde, S., Bracke, P. and Levecque, K. (2010) 'Gender differences in depression in 23 European countries. Cross-national variation in the gender gap in depression', *Social Science and Medicine*, 71(2): 305–313.

Vandoros, S., Avendano, M. and Kawachi, I. (2019) 'The association between economic uncertainty and suicide in the short-run', *Social Science and Medicine*, 220: 403–410.

Varcoe, C., Browne, A. and Blanchet Garneau, A. (2019) 'Beyond stress and coping: The relevance of critical theoretical perspectives to conceptualising racial discrimination in health research', *Health Sociology Review*, 28: 245–260.

Verhaeghe, M. and Bracke, P. (2012) 'Associative stigma among mental health professionals: Implications for professional and service user well-being', *Journal of Health and Social Behavior*, 53(1): 17–32.

Vigo, D., Kestel, D., Pendakur, K., Thornicroft, G. and Atun, R. (2019) 'Disease burden and government spending on mental, neurological, and substance use disorders, and self-harm: Cross-sectional, ecological study of health system response in the Americas', *Lancet Public Health*, 4(2): e89-e96.

Villatoro, A., Mays, V., Ponce, N. and Aneshensel, C. (2018a) 'Perceived need for mental health care: The intersection of race, ethnicity, gender, and socioeconomic status', *Society and Mental Health*, 8(1): 1–24.

Villatoro, A., Dupont-Reyes, M., Phelan, J., Painter, K. and Link, B. (2018b) 'Parental recognition of preadolescent mental health problems: Does stigma matter?', *Social Science and Medicine*, 216: 88–96.

Viney, W. (2016) 'Getting the measure of twins' in A. Whitehead, A. Woods, S. Atkinson, J. Macnaughton and J. Richards (eds) *Edinburgh Companion to the Critical Medical Humanities*, Edinburgh: University of Edinburgh Press, pp 104–119.

Viruell-Fuentes, E., Miranda, P. and Abdulrahim, S.. (2012) 'More than culture: Structural racism, intersectionality theory, and immigrant health', *Social Science and Medicine*, 75(12): 2099–2106.

Visweswaran, K. (2010) *Un/Common Cultures: Racism and the Rearticulation of Cultural Difference*, Durham, NC: Duke University Press.

Vyncke, B. and Van Gorp, B. (2020) 'Using counterframing strategies to enhance anti-stigma campaigns related to mental illness', *Social Science and Medicine*, 258: 113090.

Wadman, R., Vostanis, P., Sayal, K., Majumder, P., Harroe, C., Clarke, D., Armstrong, M. and Townsend, E. (2018) 'An interpretative phenomenological analysis of young people's self-harm in the context of interpersonal stressors and supports: Parents, peers, and clinical services', *Social Science and Medicine*, 212: 120–128.

Wallace, J. (2012) 'Mental health and stigma in the medical profession', *Health*, 16(1): 3–18.

Wang, B., Li, X., Stanton, B. and Fang, X. (2010) 'The influence of social stigma and discriminatory experience on psychological distress and quality of life among rural-to-urban migrants in China', *Social Science & Medicine*, 71(1): 84–92.

Warin, M. (2000) 'The glass cage: An ethnography of exposure in schizophrenia', *Health*, 4(1): 115–133.

Warin, M. (2010) *Abject Relations: Everyday Worlds of Anorexia*, New Brunswick, NJ: Rutgers University Press.

Warin, M., Kowal, E. and Meloni, M. (2020) 'Indigenous knowledge in a postgenomic landscape: The politics of epigenetic hope and reparation in Australia', *Science, Technology, & Human Values*, 45(1): 87–111.

Watters, E. (2010) *Crazy Like Us: The Globalization of the American Psyche*, New York, NY: Free Press.

Webb, M., Rohe, W., Nguyen, M., Frescoln, K., Donegan, M. and Han, H. (2017) 'Finding HOPE: Changes in depressive symptomology following relocation from distressed public housing', *Social Science and Medicine*, 190: 165–173.

Weber, F. (2001) 'Settings, interactions and things: A plea for multi-integrative ethnography', *Ethnography*, 2(4): 475–499.

Weber, F. (2015) *Brève Histoire de L'anthropologie*, Paris: Flammarion.

Weller, S., Baer, R., Garcia de Alba Garcia, R. and Salcedo Rocha, A. (2008) 'Susto and nervios: Expressions for stress and depression', *Culture, Medicine, and Psychiatry*, 32(3): 406–420.

Wethington, J., Almeida, D. and Wethington, E. (2004) 'Chronic stressors and daily hassles: Unique and interactive relationships with psychological distress', *Journal of Health and Social Behavior*, 45(1): 17–33.

Wexler, L. (2006) 'Inupiat youth suicide and culture loss: Changing community conversations for prevention', *Social Science and Medicine*, 63(11): 2938–2948.

Wheaton, B. (1990) 'Life transitions, role histories, and mental health', *American Sociological Review*, 55(2): 209–223.

Wheaton, B. (2007) 'The twain meet: Distress, disorder and the continuing conundrum of categories (comment on Horwitz)', *Health*, 11(2): 303–319.

Whitaker, R. (2011) *Anatomy of an Epidemic: Psychiatric Drugs and the Astonishing Rise of Mental Illness in America*, New York, NY: Crown.

Whitley, R. and Campbell, R. (2014) 'Stigma, agency and recovery amongst people with severe mental illness', *Social Science and Medicine*, 107: 1–8.

Whooley, O. (2010) 'Diagnostic ambivalence: psychiatric workarounds and the Diagnostic and Statistical Manual of Mental Disorders', *Sociology of Health and Illness*, 32(3): 452–469.

Whooley, O. (2019) *On the Heels of Ignorance: Psychiatry and the Politics of Not Knowing*, Chicago, IL: University of Chicago Press.

Whynacht, A. (2018) 'Marks on bodies: Agential cuts as felt experience', Catalyst: Feminism, *Theory, Technoscience*, 4(1): 1–30.

Widger, T. (2012) 'Suffering, frustration, and anger: Class, gender and history in Sri Lankan suicide stories', *Culture Medicine, and Psychiatry*, 36(2): 225–244.

Wilkinson, R. and Pickett, K. (2009) *The Spirit Level: Why Equality is Better for Everyone*, London: Penguin.

Williams, A., Sarker, M. and Ferdous, S. (2018) 'Cultural attitudes toward postpartum depression in Dhaka, Bangladesh', *Medical* Anthropology, 37(3): 194–205.

Williams, D. (2018) 'Stress and the mental health of populations of color: Advancing our understanding of race-related stressors', *Journal of Health and Social Behavior*, 59(4): 466–485.

Williams, S. and Bendelow, G. (1998) *The Lived Body: Sociological Themes, Embodied Issues*, London: Routledge.

Williams, T., Davis, J., Figueira, C. and Vizard, T. (2021) 'Coronavirus and depression in adults, Great Britain: January to March 2021' *Office of National Statistics National Bulletin*, 5 May. Available from: www.ons.gov.uk/peoplepopulationandcommunity/wellbeing/articles/coronavirusanddepressioninadultsgreatbritain/januarytomarch2021 [Accessed 30 November 2021]

Wolfe, P. (2016) *Traces of History: Elementary Structures of Race*, London: Verso Books.

Woodgate, R., Comaskey, B., Tennent, P., Wener, P. and Altman, G. (2020) 'The wicked problem of stigma for youth living with anxiety', *Qualitative Health Research*, 30(10): 1491–1502.

World Health Organization (WHO) (2020) *Mental Health Atlas 2020*, Geneva: WHO.

Wouters, C. (2007) *Informalization: Manners and Emotions Since 1890*, London: Sage.

Wright, A., Jorm, A. and Mackinnon, A. (2011) 'Labeling of mental disorders and stigma in young people', *Social Science & Medicine*, 73(4):498–506.

X, T. and polanco, M. (2021) 'An autopsy of the coloniality of suicide: Modernity's completed genocide', *Health*, 13634593211038517.

Yang, J. (2016) 'The politics and regulation of anger in urban China', *Culture, Medicine and Psychiatry*, 40(1): 100–123.

Yeshua-Katz, D. (2015) 'Online stigma resistance in the pro-ana community', *Qualitative Health Research*, 25(10): 1347–1358.

Yildiz, U. (2016) '"Precarity" of the territorialized state: Immigrants re-drawing and re-mapping the borders', *Journal of Borderlands Studies*, 31(4): 521–536.

Youdell, D., Harwood, V. and Lindley, M. (2018) 'Biological sciences, social sciences and the languages of stress', *Discourse: Studies in the Cultural Politics of Education*, 39(2): 219–241.

Young, R., Sweeting, H. and West, P. (2006) 'Prevalence of deliberate self-harm and attempted suicide within contemporary Goth youth subculture: Longitudinal cohort study', *BMJ*, 332: 1058–1061.

Younis, T. and Jadhav, S. (2020) 'Islamophobia in the National Health Service: An ethnography of institutional racism in PREVENT's counter-radicalisation policy', *Sociology of Health and Illness*, 42(3), 610–626.

Yu, Y. and Williams, D. (1999) 'Socioeconomic status and mental health' in C. Aneshensel and J. Phelan (eds) *Handbook of the Sociology of Mental Health*, New York, NY: Springer, pp 151–166.

Yue, E. (2021) 'Migrant suicide: A case for intersectional suicide research', *Journal Of Ethics In Mental Health*, 11(10): online.

Zerubavel, E. (1997) *Social Mindscapes: An Invitation to Cognitive Sociology*, Cambridge, MA: Harvard University Press.

Zola, I. (1972) 'Medicine as an institution of social control', *The Sociological Review*, 20(4): 487–504.

Index

References to endnotes show the page number, note number and chapter number (136n8(ch2)).

A
Abrutyn, S. 17, 104
African American communities 58
African Americans 14, 31, 32, 52, 53, 54, 60
age 15, 17–18
agency 74–77
Alang, S.M. 31–32, 58
Alexander, J. 109
allostatic load 40
Allouch, A. 26
amplification model 101, 108
anger 57–60, 125
Angermeyer, M.C. 78
anorexia 26–17, 57, 99–100, 100–101
Anthropocene 110
anthropological-discursive paradigm 111
anti-psychiatric movement 108, 127
anxiety 25, 26, 118–119, 120
Archaeology of Knowledge (Foucault) 69
Armstrong, D. 69, 70
artefact explanations 19
associative stigma 78
Atatürk, M.K. 109
Atkinson, S. 124
attention deficit hyperactivity disorder (ADHD) 12, 56, 119
attribution theory 79
autism 29, 32, 82, 83, 101
autism epidemics 81, 120

B
Balandier, G. 94
Balland, L. 25
Baller, R. 17
Barbee, H. 73
Barnard, A. 82
Barrett, A. 47
Barrett, R.J. 74
Basic Problems in Ethnopsychiatry (Devereux) 95
Bateson, G. 95, 96
Beam, C. 39–40

Bearman, P. 83
behavioural explanations 19
Behrouzan, O. 98
Being Mentally Ill (Scheff) 66–67
Benedict, R. 93–94, 101
Berlin Wall 108–109
Besseling, B. 84
Best, J. 61
Billaud, J. 110
bio-psycho-social models 111–112
biology 40–41
biomedicine 97
bipolar disorder 18, 119, 130
Bipolar Expeditions (Martin) 101
Birth of the Clinic (Foucault) 69
black men 57
black people 14
   see also African Americans; people of colour
Black Report 12
Black Skin, White Masks (Fanon) 94
Blackdog Institute 119
Blazer, D. 3
Boas, F. 93
Bonniau, B. 83
Bonnin, J.E. 75
borderline personality disorder 76
Borovoy, A. 100
Bourdieu, P. 24, 128
Bourgois, P. 59
Bowleg, L. 21
Braedley, S. 30
Brinkmann, S. 85
Bröer, C. 84
Brossard, B. 27, 113, 121
Brothers Karamazov (Dostoevsky) 90, 115
Brown, T.N. 106
burnout 102
Busfield, J. 72, 87

C
Canguihelm, G. 69
Cant, S. 26

INDEX

capitalism 87
capitalist colonialism 93
Carde, E. 22
Castel, F. 70
Castel, P.-E. 56
categories 65, 80–83
  see also labelling theories
categorization, politics of 71–79
  labels in everyday life 74–77
  legitimacy of labels 72–74
  stigma 77–79
categorization processes 7
causality hypothesis 18
Center for Epidemiologic Studies Depression Scale (CES-D) 31–32
Chamak, B. 83
Chandler, A. 24, 51, 52, 86
Cheslack-Postava, K. 32
Chua, J.L. 75
city life 36–37
civilising processes 57
class 11, 12, 16, 28, 31, 41–42
class neurosis 26
classifications 65
  see also labelling theories
Cohen, B. 29–30, 122
cohorts 18
collaborations 39, 40–42
Collins, P.Y. 23
colonial dynamics 130
colonial governance 92–93
colonialism 114
coloniality 114
colonization 94–95
community studies 10–11
compassionate ethos 128
conditions of possibility 102
configuration 25, 136n11(ch1)
configurational perspectives 10, 24–27, 120
Conrad, P. 72–73, 87
conspiracy theories 61
context 20, 45–46
contradictory class locations 13–14
Cooper, D. 60
coping resources 46, 47
correlation, paradigm of 19–20, 21
cortisol 40, 44, 62
cortisol sociology 111–112
COVID-19 61, 118, 120
critical phenomenology 24
critical realism 72
Csordas, T. 57–58, 84–85
cultural competence 106
cultural consonance model 104, 130
cultural contradiction 103
cultural explanations 19, 92–96
cultural expression 107–110
cultural loss model 105
cultural objects 108–109

cultural polarity 113, 132
cultural trauma 109
culture 90–92, 127, 130–132
  contemporary perspectives 105–107
  integrative models 110–115
  within people 103–105
  people within 100–102
"culture and personality" school 93–94
culture-bound syndromes 98, 99
culture clash 103, 130

D

Darmon, M. 26–27
De Gaulejac, V. 26
death-consciousness 98
decolonial approaches 113–115
deficit narrative 108
definitional perspectives 10, 27–32, 122
Dein, S. 102
deinstitutionalization 82
demand-side perspectives 81
Dengah, H. 104
depoliticization 87
depression
  and anger 58
  and culture 91, 97, 98, 99, 101–102
  and family forms 47
  and gender 15, 28–29
  labelling theories 66, 75
  and medicalization 57
  prevalence 118–119, 120, 130
  and socioeconomic status 12
deprivation 120
Devereux, G. 95
deviance 104
diagnosis 84–85, 86–88, 127, 129
  attention deficit hyperactivity disorder (ADHD) 12
  autism 32, 81
  bias in 14
  depression 66
  and local settings 74–76
  and self-labelling 68
Diagnostic and Statistical Manual of Mental Disorders (DSM) 135n1(ch1)
  anger 57
  culture-bound syndromes 98, 99
  delusional states 31
  gendered and productivist expectations 122
  labelling 65
  paranoia 60, 62
  self-injury 86
  sex addiction 81
  symptoms 29–30
diagnostic processes 83
diffusion model 100, 101
disadvantaged racial groups 14
Discipline and Punish (Foucault) 69
discourse 107

discrimination 22–23, 26, 53–54
discursive resemblances 102
dissociative experiences 111
dissonant combinations 22
distress 25–26, 31, 45, 49
Donovan, R. 23
double absence 103
double blind theory of schizophrenia 95
Dressler, W. 104, 112
Dudgeon, P. 114
Dunham, H. 11
dynamic nominalism 72

E

eating disorders *see* anorexia
ecological niches 112–113, 131
ecosophical praxis of care 114
educational attainment 12, 17
Ehrenberg, A. 101–102
Elias, N. 56, 57
embodiment model 32, 85–86
Emerson, R. 68
emotional expression 31–32, 49
emotional isolation 103
emotional repression 56
emotions 50–51, 53, 93, 125
   sociology of 55–62
Enjolras, F. 3
environmental crisis 110
environmental factors 3
epidemics 113
   see also autism epidemics
Epidemiologic Catchment Area Study 11
episteme 69
Epstein-Barr virus 112
ethnic minorities 52
ethnicity 14, 20, 23, 52, 106
   see also African Americans
ethno-psychiatry 95
Europe 119
evasion 132
expatriates 61
Eyal, G. 81, 82

F

family 15, 25, 27, 47
   family forms 47
Fanon, F. 87, 94–95
Faris, R. 11
Fassin, D. 61, 70–71, 88, 128
Fisher, M. 35
Flood, M. 30
Fong, V. 25
Foucault, M. 6, 7, 65, 66, 69–71, 83–84, 107
France 20
Frankfurt School 55
Friberg, T. 74
Friedman, J. 82
Friedman, S. 26

G

gender 15, 28–29, 30, 38, 50–52, 122, 124–125
   see also men; women
gender dysphoria 76
generational mobility 17
generosity 81
genes 112
genetics 39–40
geopolitical dynamics 106–107
German psychology 108–109
global mental health 96, 130
Goffman, E. 77, 88
Goldstein, M. 67–68
Gove, W. 67
governmentality 70–71
Graeber, D. 107
Grinker, R. 129
Guerin, B. 88
Gulbas, L. 103

H

Hacking, I. 4, 71, 72, 85, 112–113, 131
Haldol 57
hallucinations 88–89
Han, B.-C. 102
Harper, D. 31, 61–62
Hirshbein, L. 28–29, 31–32
History of Madness (Foucault) 69
History of Sexuality (Foucault) 69
Hollingshead, A. 11, 28
Holman, D. 28
honour suicide 106
Horn, J. 114
Horwitz, A. 44, 49–50, 111
hysteresis 26

I

identity-salient stressors 54
Illich, I. 87
immigration health paradox 17
individualization 87
inequalities in mental health 10–21, 28–29, 120–123
   age 17–18
   explanatory models 18–21
      alternative perspectives 21–32
   gender 15, 28–29
   LGBT+ people 15–16
   marital status 15
   migrants 17
   neighbourhoods 16
   racial groups 14
   social mobility 17
   social networks 16–17
   socioeconomic status (SES) 10–14
injustice 59, 121
integrative models 131
inter- and intra-generational social mobility 17

INDEX

interdisciplinary work 39, 40–42
intersectional perspectives 10, 21–24, 49, 120–121
inversion model 101–102

J
Jackson, M. 43
Jadhev, S. 88
Jaworski, K. 30
Jenkins, J. 56, 57–58, 84–85
Johnson, A. 76
Jordon-Young, R.M. 32

K
Kaiser, N. 23
Kapp, S. 108
Karlsson, M. 23
Katzman, M. 27, 101
Kawachi, I. 13, 121
King, M. 83
Kirmayer, L. 111
Kitanka, J. 76–77
Kleinman, A. 98, 99
Kohn, M. 16

L
labelling theories 7, 65, 66–69, 126–129, 137n2(ch3)
  function of labels 86–89
  labels in everyday life 74–77
  legitimacy of labels 72–74
  madness 69–71
  performativity of language 83–86
  socio-political arrangements 80–83
  stigma 77–79
Lareau, M. 41–42
Lee, M. 13, 121
legitimation 74
Lemert, E. 61
Leonard Pearlin Award 56, 136n8(ch2)
Lester, R. 100, 105
Leuenberger, C. 108
LGBT+ people 15–16, 53–54
Link, B. 67, 68
Littlewood, R. 100, 102
Longest, K. 51, 52
looping effects 85, 112
Luhrmann, T. 105
Lui, M. 27
Luna Sánchez, S.E. 114
Lupton, D. 56
Lutz, C. 99

M
Madame Bovary (Flaubert) 9, 10, 21
madness 69–71, 78, 90, 92, 97, 108, 131
Marcuse, H. 55
marital status 15
marriage 39–40
materialist explanations 19

Maturo, F. 73
Mauss, M. 93
Maynard, D. 74, 82
McDade, T. 112
McEwen, C. and B. 40, 41–42, 46, 58
McLeod, J. 44, 46, 62
McMahon, R. 85
McWade, B. 108, 111–112
Mead, M. 94
medical colonization 87
medical naturalism 71–72
Medical Nemesis (Illich) 87
medical taxonomy 112, 131
medicalization processes 72–74, 81
men 15, 28–29, 32, 39–40, 50–51, 54
mental health
  definition 29–30
mental health apparatus 3
mental health categories 84
mental health crisis 118–120, 125
Mental Health Foundation 118, 123
mental health inequalities 10–21, 120–123
  age 17–18
  explanatory models 18–21
    alternative perspectives 21–32
  marital status 15
  neighbourhoods 16
  social mobility 17
  social networks 16–17
  socioeconomic status (SES) 10–14
mental health professionals 28, 29
Messinger, S. 68
Metzl, J. 57, 60
Meyer, I. 53–54
micro-politics of trouble 68–69
Migliore, S. 84
migrants 22–23, 38, 43, 106
migration 17, 103
minority stress 16, 35, 49, 53–55, 124
Mirdamadi, M. 98
Mirowsky, J. 61, 87
modes of production 13
modified labelling theory 68
Mora-Rios, J. 22
moral conservatism 46–48
Moreau, N. 102
Moreno Pestaña, J.-L. 113
Moretti, V. 73
Morrall, P. 2
Mueller, A. 17, 104
Multicultural Mental Health Australia 99
Murat, L. 87, 109

N
Näckter, S. 23
Nakamura, K. 88–89
National Intelligence Council (NIC), US 117, 125
neighbourhoods 16, 38

191

neoliberal subjectivation 124
neoliberal turn 123–124
neurodiversity 108, 110
neuroscience 3
  neuro-biochemical 31
  neuro-biological 40–42
  neurochemistry 42
Ng, E. 18, 101
Nishimura, J. 12
North African Syndrome 95

O
observability 113, 131
Oedipus complex 94–95
Order of Things (Foucault) 69
O'Reilly, M. 74
Orr, J. 57
Ortega, F. 108
Owens, J. 12
Oyarce Pisani, A.M. 114

P
panic disorders 57
paradigm of correlation 19–20, 21
paradox of paranoia 61
paranoia 31, 60–62, 125
parenting styles 41–42
pathogenic social mobility 17
Pearlin, L. 35
Pearson, V. 27
people of colour 31, 62
  see also black people
performativity of language 83–86
pharmaceutical industry 73, 96
Pickett, K. 121
Picone, M. 106
Pietila, I. 43
Pike, K. 100
Pilgrim, D. 4, 71–72
political devices, diagnosis as 88
political unrest 59
politics of categorization 71–79
  labels in everyday life 74–77
  legitimacy of labels 72–74
  stigma 77–79
Pollner, M. 67
population studies 11
post-traumatic stress disorder (PTDS) 81, 104, 114, 119
postcolonial approaches 113–115
poverty 10–11, 43, 46, 55, 120
power 69–70
  see also social domination
power dynamics 56
Price-Robertson, R. 25
Prickett, P. 84
Pringle, Y. 114
Prins, S. 13
Prior, P. 30
production, modes of 13

psy-
  psy-categories 127
  psy-discourses 3, 71, 96
  psy-professionals 30
  psy-professions 70, 81
psychiatric
  hegemony 30
  paradox 2–3
psychiatric-adaptive paradigm 111
psychiatry 70, 76–77, 80–81, 87, 94–95, 97, 114
psychic disability 82
psychology 70, 81–82, 93, 96, 97, 108–109
psychosis 36–37, 42, 109

R
race 14, 20, 52–53, 124
race mental health paradox 14
racial bias 14
racial groups 14
racial minorities 52
racism 57
radical constructivism 72
radical relativist position 99
Rahimi, S. 109
re-formalization 129
realism 4
  see also medical naturalism
Rechtman, R. 88
Redlich, F. 11, 28
Rees, S. 59
relative status 13
repressive surplus 55
Richards, D. 61
Richardson, K. 17
River, J. 30
Roberts, C. 62, 111–112
Rogers, A. 4
Rose, N. 70, 71, 81, 87, 108
Ross, C. 61, 87
Russia 115–116
Rytkonen, M. 43

S
Sakit Hati 59
Sakurai, K. 13
Satariano, B. 18
Sayad, A. 103
Scambler, G. 88
Scheff, T. 7, 65, 66–67, 71, 137n2(ch3)
Scheper-Hughes, N. 25, 95–96
Schieman, S. 56
schizophrenia
  configurational perspectives 25
  and culture 109
  double blind theory 95–96
  intersectional perspectives 22
  and paranoia 60
  prevalence 130

INDEX

and religion 102
and urbanization 16
Schneider, J. 72–73, 87
Schnittker, J. 39
Schulze, B. 78
Schwartz, O. 43
Schwartz, S. 44, 46
Scull, A. 71
selection hypothesis 18
self-harm / self-injury 5
 and bodily practices 86
 and sexuality 16
 and social positioning 27
 and stress 51–52
 white working class men 24
 young women 103, 125
self-labelling 68
self-salience theory 15
Seligman, R. 111
Selye, H. 37, 46
Sepúlveda Jara, R. 114
sex addiction 73, 74, 81
sex role theory 15
Shorer, S. 104
Silve, D. 59
Simmel, G. 36
Simon, R. 50, 54
Simopoulou, Z. 51
Slater, T. 88
Snedker, K.A. 89
social capital 16–17, 18
social cases 82
social class 11, 12, 16, 28, 31, 41–42
social constructivism 4
social determinants 10–14
social domination 49–55
social drift hypothesis 18
social inequalities 49–55
social isolation 16
social isolation stress disorder 125
social justice 33
 see also injustice
social mobility 11, 17, 26, 27
social networks 16–17
social organization of trust 61–62
social positions 6, 9–10
 configurational perspectives 24–27, 120
 correlational perspective 10–21
 definitional perspectives 27–32, 122
 intersectional perspectives 21–24, 120–121
 socialization to emotions 53
social role explanations 19
social stratification 6–7
social transformation 88
socio-political arrangements 80–83, 127
socioeconomic status (SES) 11–13, 16
sociology of emotions 55–62
sociology of mental health 2–4, 8, 45–46, 133

Sorokin's dissociative thesis 17
Souza Prado, G.A. 114
"Special Initiative for Mental Health" (WHO) 130
specialization 8, 80, 89, 132
Spleen 100
split-relativist position 98
Srole, L. 11
status incongruence 13
Steggals, P. 102, 110
stigma 54–55, 68, 77–79, 88, 127
stress 112
 and social domination 49–55
 social origins 36–37
 see also minority stress
stress explanations 19
stress paradigm 7, 34–49, 60, 123–126
 biological origin 39–42
 limitations and problems 42–49
stress process model 35, 55
structural resemblances 102
subcultures 106
subjective status 13
suicide 5
 cultural consonance model 104
 cultural loss model 105
 and emotional isolation 103
 and gender 15, 30, 51–52, 110
 honour suicide 106
 and neighbourhoods 16, 17
 prevalence 119, 125
 and race/ethnicity 20
 and social positioning 27
Sri Lanka 23–24
Summerfield, D. 99
surveillance 31, 62
surveillance medicine 70
Sweet, E. 124

T
Takeuchi, D. 106
Tan, C. 76
Taylor, C. 40
thinking processes 109–110
Thoits, P. 42, 45, 51, 52, 54, 67, 68
threshold 113
"total man" 93
Townsend, P. 12
Tran, A. 75
transcultural psychiatry 91
transgender people 76
transgressions 66–67, 93
transient mental illness 112
trauma 30–31, 41, 107
 cultural 109
treatment gap 128
trust 61–62
Tseris, E. 30–31
Turner, B. 114

Turner, J. 47
Turner, R. 50, 58
Turowetz, J. 74, 83
Tyler, I. 88

U

United Kingdom (UK)
  COVID-19 118, 120
  mental health crisis 125
  mental illness prevalence 118–119
  race 20
  racial bias 14
  research projects 5
  stress 123
United States (US)
  mental illness prevalence 119–120
  National Intelligence Council (NIC) 117, 125
  race 20
  race mental health paradox 14
  research projects 5
  stressful dominations 53
universalist position 97
unmet needs 128
urbanization 36
US National Comorbidity Study 11

V

Veronika Decides to Die (Coelho) 34, 63
Vigo, D. 126
Viruell-Fuentes, E. 22

W

Walker, R. 114
Warin, M. 85
Watters, E. 99
Weber, F. 25
wellbeing 114
West, L. 23
Wexler, L. 105
Widger, T. 23
Wilkinson, R. 121
Williams, D. 44
Woman on the Edge of Time (Piercy) 64, 89
women
  depression 28–29
  emotional expression 32
  safety 31
  stress 39–40, 50–51, 54
  suicide 15, 30
  surveillance 62
World Health Organization 96, 119, 130
Wouters, C. 129

Y

Yang, J. 59, 60
Younis, T. 88

Z

Zayas, L. 103